BONES & BREAKS

Total Orthopaedic Solutions

Dr Sushil Sharma

VitaMed
An Imprint of
Vitasta Publishing Pvt Ltd

Published by
Renu Kaul Verma
Vitasta Publishing Pvt Ltd
2/15, Ansari Road, Daryaganj
New Delhi - 110 002
info@vitastapublishing.com

Consulting Editors:

Dr Vikas Bharadwaj
MS, DNB (Ortho)

Dr Mohit Madan
MS, MCh (Ortho)
Spl Sports Injury

ISBN 978-93-86473-01-1

Cover and layout by Vits Press
Printed by Vikas Computer and Printers

To my mother Maya Devi, for having a belief that everybody can contribute positively in life. Also, to millions of patients who fight and win over illness.

Acknowledgements

First of all I greatly acknowledge my teachers who transferred their knowledge of specific subjects to me which I could share with people.

Thanks to our young consultants Dr Vikas Bharadwaj and Dr Mohit Madan for their useful inputs before finalisation of the manuscript.

Many thanks to Sunny Mehra for his continuous and untiring support. Thanks to Kailash Jain, Trustee Secretary AFI, for all the encouragement.

Last but not the least, my best friend, confidant, wife and trustee AFI, Dr Seema Sharma for making everything possible.

Foreword

Awareness about musculoskeletal ailments is a big issue all over the world and more so in developing countries like India. AFI and its chairman, Dr Sushil Sharma, are doing a wonderful job by educating the masses through a short, easy to understand book in the form of Q & A on topics like arthritis, osteoporosis, factures, bone tumours, sports injuries, developmental problems etc. Needless to say that the descriptions in the book are very reader friendly. I am very optimistic about the response the book will generate from people; we will consider if the book can be translated and used for awareness of masses in other countries as well.

Prof Jean-Yves Reginster
President ESCEO and
Board member IOF, Belgium

Foreword

Bones & Breaks: Total Orthopaedic Solutions is an innovative and absorbing treatise which endeavours to simplify the complex orthopaedic conditions and their management by describing them as FAQs. The questions (124 in all distributed over 13 chapters) describe real life scenarios and are addressed in a generalised though realistic manner. Abundant illustrations render the understanding of complex anatomy and its pathological disruption easy. The last three chapters dealing with Physiotherapy, Yoga and Gymming are a must read for avid fans of physical fitness with pearls of Dos and Don'ts provided with relation to various gymming equipment. Overall, Dr Sushil Sharma and Arthritis Foundation of India have done a great job of providing an easy to read and understand book on Orthopaedic Solutions which will prove a very useful tool for public education and awareness.

Dr Rajesh Malhotra
MS, FRCS, FACS, FICS, FIMSA, MNASc
Professor & Head, Department of Orthopaedics, AIIMS, New Delhi

Contents

Preface

It's a fact that a majority of patients are not able to understand the complex musculoskeletal problems confronting them.

Orthopaedic surgeons keep struggling with patients in order to make them understand their specific kind of bone and muscle ailments broadly for smooth treatment.

During the process of clearing doubts, the 'Frequently Asked Questions' format was unanimously considered most effective and to the point, and therefore, this format has been chosen for dissemination of relevant information for this book.

Our idea at the Arthritis Foundation of India was to educate curious citizens who want to know and learn about bones, joints and related muscles along with arthritis. Also provide an easy to use side table book for general practitioner doctors who usually don't get time to revise basic orthopaedics.

Hope this book serves this twin purpose in a stimulating and easily understood way.

Trauma & Fractures

Q1: My aunt who is in her 60s fell in the dining room and injured her right shoulder. Now she can't lift her arm. Doctor says that she needs a surgery. Is it a serious issue?

Fracture at the upper end of the arm bone (around the shoulder) is a very common consequence after a fall. A fracture with one line (ie. in 2 parts—head and shaft) can be managed with plaster but 3 or 4

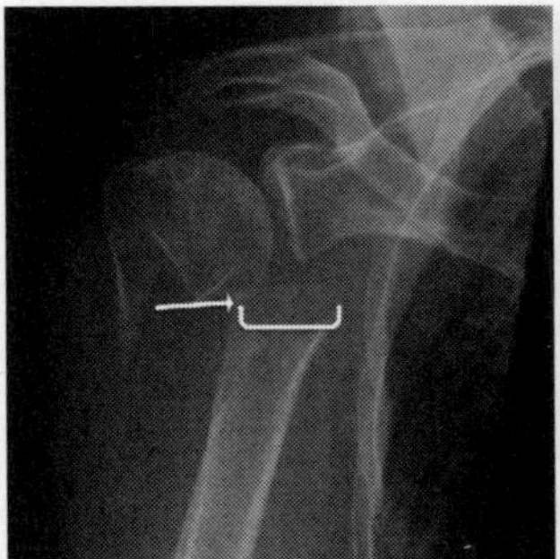

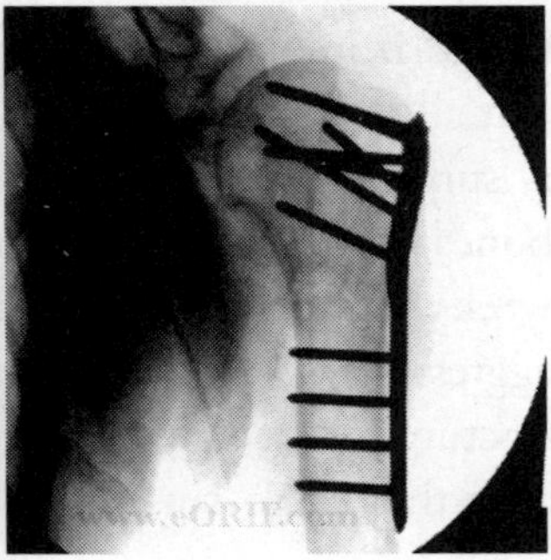

parts fracture of upper end of arm bone may need surgery (correct positioning and fixation with plate). This kind of surgery helps in union of fracture in about 6-8 weeks and also allows early movements which are important to avoid stiff shoulder. Usually multiple part fractures in young patients happen with severe trauma but in elderly women like your aunt, it can happen with trivial injury because of weak bones (osteoporosis). Well, in all cases, post surgery physiotherapy is of immense value.

Q2: I had a scooter accident and broke my collar bone. The casualty medical officer of the government hospital has given me just a shoulder arm pouch, is it sufficient? I doubt.

The collar bone is a very commonly fractured bone and old school of orthopedics says 90-95% of fracture clavicle unite with a 'Clavicle figure of eight belt', and nothing more is required. The time of union is usually 6 weeks and normally on X-Rays the horizontal fracture ends are overriding each other. But all that is acceptable.

A surgery is only indicated in selected cases, when bones don't unite and remain painful even after 6-8 weeks, where the bony spike is impinging the skin aggressively. Also when the lateral end of the clavicle fractures, which are likely to create functional deficit after the not-so-correct healing.

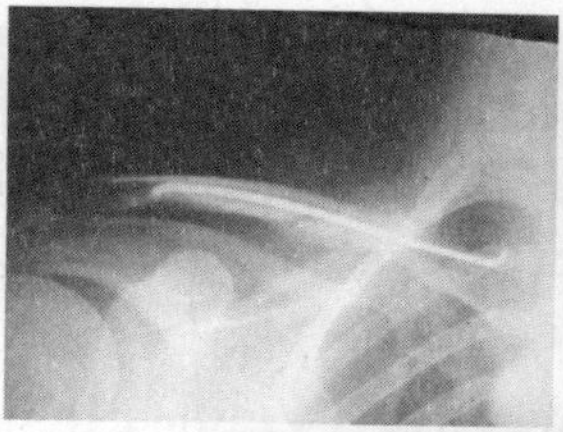

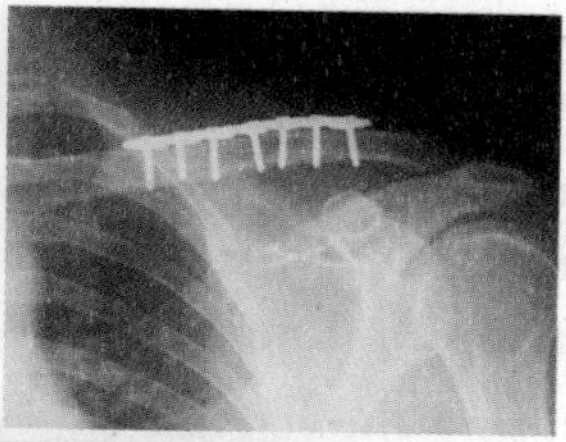

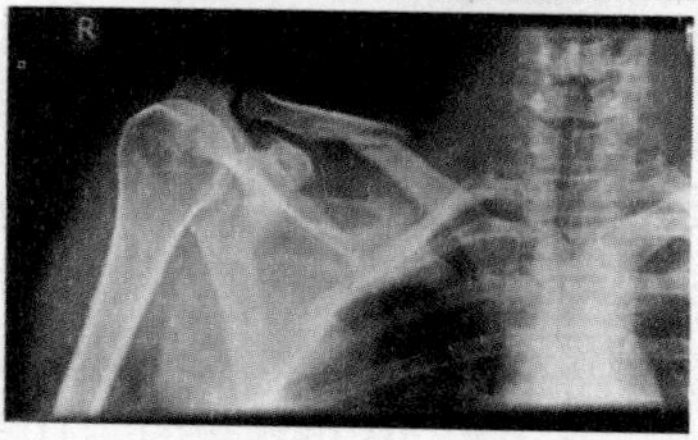

There are pre-contoured plates available for clavicle fractures if surgery is required. Some small outer end fresh fractures can be fixed percutaneously with steel wires too, with plate and K wire fixation.

Q3: Once I watched a child's index finger chopped off with a sharp knife. Can the finger, which is completely detached from the body, be reattached?

Looks unlikely. In cases of fingers, micro vascular surgery is not easy and the success rate is very low but the same is not true about bigger limbs like forearm and leg where plastic and vascular surgeons can do a good job. Nevertheless, plastic and vascular surgeons are capable of saving the fingers sometimes, provided the patient is operated within 4 to 6 hours after the trauma.

Q4: I am a paramedic at a Primary Health Center (PHC) in a rural subdivision and we get quite a few cases of injuries of crushed hands (from crusher machines) which we refer to higher centers. I am curious to know what their fate is.

During the harvest season thresher-crushed injuries are common in villages which lead to mutilation of hands, may be of the forearm too. Besides the bones, tendons (the muscles elongations), nerves (for sensation) and blood vessels (for blood supply) are also damaged and to salvage the limb/hand, blood supply needs to be restored first. This has to be followed by treatment of other components to make the limb functional. This is a very uphill task and needs joint effort of vascular, plastic and orthopedic surgeons. May take a long time for rehabilitation.

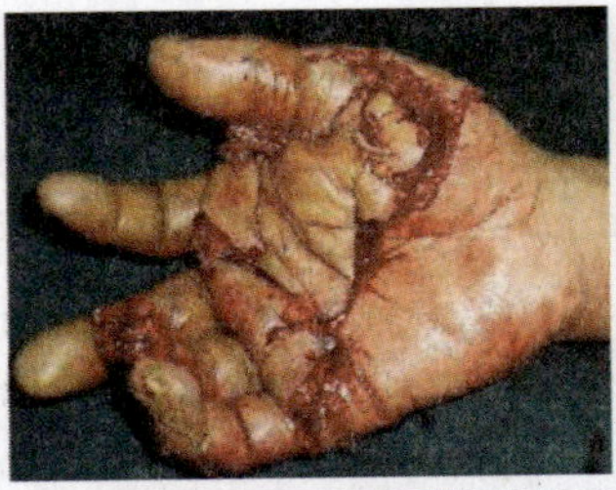

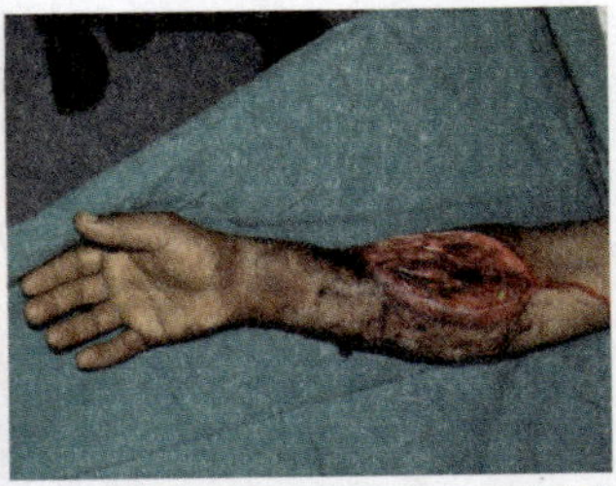

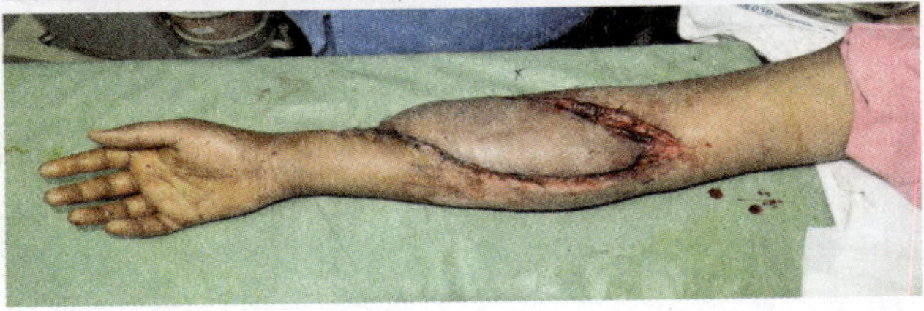

Q5: My son is a young charted accountant and sustained fracture of arm, which was operated upon. But even after the fracture healing, the wrist and hand is paralysed. Can you tell me why?

Your surprise is genuine because fracture of arm bone humerus is geographically far from wrist and fingers. Try and understand the fact that fracture of humerus (arm bone) at middle 1/3 usually needs open reduction (setting of the bone with surgery) and internal fixation by a steel or titanium plate. It can also be fixed along the medullary cavity (the hollow space in the bone) from upper to lower end by steel or titanium nail.

Once the fracture is nicely fixed, it 'most probably' will unite but alongside the bone, there is the radial nerve which provides strength (motor supply) to muscles of wrist and hand. Any injury to this nerve by the fractured fragments preoperatively or during surgery results in the loss of stretching movement of the hand upwards. Your son may have suffered something of this type.

In such a case, your son needs to wait for 6-8 weeks and then go for a special test called Nerve Conduction Velocity (NCV) test and EMG (Electromyography) test to ascertain the seriousness of injury. The orthopedic surgeon may ask you to wait and watch for natural recovery and if unfortunately it doesn't happen, the option is either repair of the nerve and if this is not possible, other muscle tendons are transferred to compensate for the paralysed group of muscle. Both the surgeries are technically demanding but in expert hands the results are satisfactory.

Q6: My son is only 8 years old and broke his long bone of thigh at the middle. The doctor gave me an option: either to go for plaster or nailing. It's very confusing. Please elaborate.

Long bone like Tibia (main bone in leg), Radius and Ulna (in forearm), Humerus (in arm) and Femur (in thigh) can be treated without any surgery in children up to 8-9 years. All they use is close setting/reduction and POP (Plaster of Paris) or fiber cast.

Anybody beyond 15-16 years has to be compulsorily operated upon because the bones can't be held in correct position and have tendency to go for non-union.

The remaining in between age group (from 8 to 16) is a grey area with no hard and fast rules and depends from case to case and doctor. For such patient, Titanium Elastic Nail (TENs) system is available now, which is introduced into the long bone from one end to other, fixing the fracture under vision, ie. computer screen guidance (image intensifier control). The surgical time is short, almost no blood loss and there is no chance of fracture displacement. So TENs is presently a good way out for this age group of children who are not adults but have large bones. You may discuss with your specialist and decide.

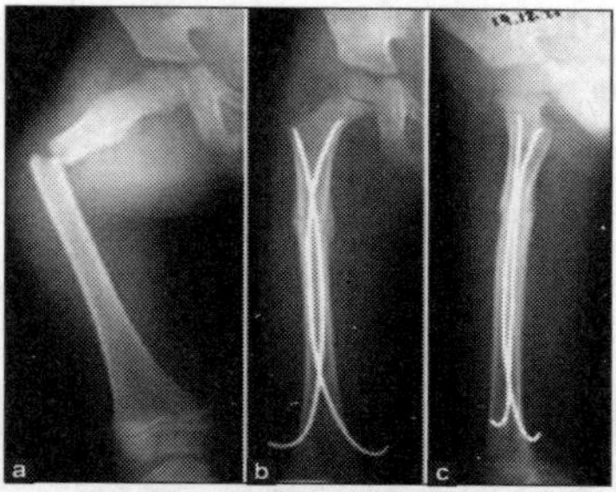

TEN nails in thigh bone (Femur)

Q7: Three months ago my aunt, 58, had a fracture at the wrist and she became alright after 2 months of plaster. Now my friend, who is just 25, sustained fracture at the same site and the doctor says it needs plate fixation. I have heard, fracture healing is difficult in the old, then why this strange advice?

The common fracture at wrist (lower end of forearm bone called radius) giving rise to dinner fork like deformity is called Colle's fracture; usually a result of osteoporosis (weak bones). Such kind of fracture in your aunt's case needed close manipulation and plaster under sedation or local anesthesia. The fracture heals in six to eight weeks; wrist exercises follow for say two weeks.

But in a young person like your friend, it is not a fragility fracture and mostly fracture fragments are displaced with involvement of wrist joint (called dorsal or Volar Barton). Although such fractures can also be close reduced and plastered, it may have residual stiffness of wrist post healing. Therefore special plates are used to surgically fix the fracture and this to follow with early mobilisation (movement) of wrist for better results. This may be the reason for the surgical advice in your friend's case. If you have any doubt, take a second opinion.

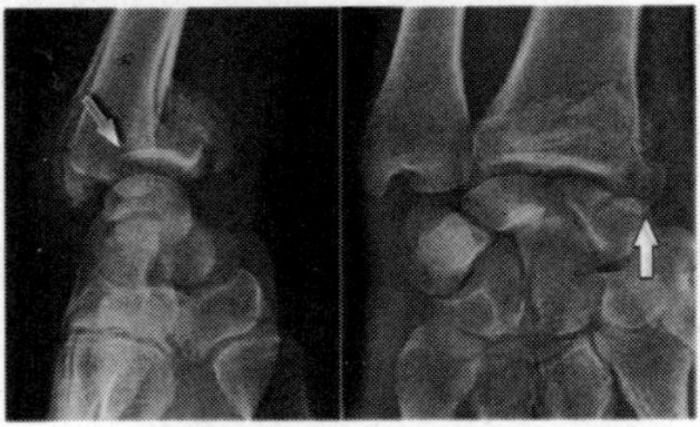

Barton's fracture

Q8: After a motorbike skid I had an injury on my fingers, doctor took an X-ray and said, it's just a soft tissue injury. Now after a month, there is deformity in 2 fingers and I can't straighten them.

First of all soft tissue injuries in fingers are not to be taken casually. You must consult an orthopedic specialist immediately because one month is a long time for finger injuries. In your case, it appears that the extension apparatus (tendon and sheath) at the back of fingers, which is required to straighten the fingers, was broken, and since the fingers were not immobilised in a straight position for one month, the tendon couldn't heal. The free pull of palmer side tendon on finger joint is responsible for bending of finger (flexion) and hence the deformity. This is buttonhole deformity, similarly mallet finger can happen at the distal end of the finger.

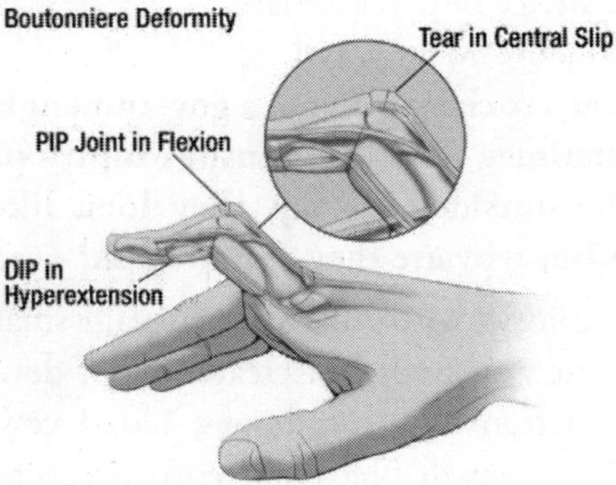

Photo of mallet finger

Now in your case, after one month, surgery is the only option. That is, open repair of extensor apparatus and fixing of the finger with straight 1mm needle-like wire, holding it in this position for one month. For sure, fingers can be salvaged but sometimes results may not be fantastic. The option is worth trying.

Q9: My friend, an IT engineer, had a bad road accident and as a result multiple fractures in body. Despite good physical recovery he is mentally not OK, why?

The problem with your friend is not rare and can happen in such circumstances. Basically it is post-traumatic stress syndrome, whereby the psychological status and behavior of sufferers get grossly disturbed.

Such patients along with physical rehabilitation also require mental rehabilitation. Best tools are counseling, psychotherapy and sometimes medicines with the advice of psychiatrist.

Q10: I am a social worker at a government hospital and sometimes there are gunshot injury patients. From the outside, per say, they look like other patients but why are they at more risk?

Gunshot injuries with bullets have usually small or not so large entry wounds but create lots of devastation and destruction of tissue, bones, blood vessels and nerves. Gun powder has very corrosive action and many wounds get infected. The damage to bones, tissues, muscles and nerve needs to be addressed on its merits but additional factors may delay the recovery. Many such patients land up with amputations.

Q11: My neighbour Antony, who works in a warehouse, has sustained injury in the right foot after a fall of heavy weight on it. Instead of reducing the swelling and treating the fractures at the hospital, the doctors gave two long cuts on the top of the foot. Why this further mutilation?

Mr Antony's foot must have been acutely swollen due to crushing of tissues and factures of the bones. Usually in such a situation blood flow in the blood vessels becomes jeopardised. This is called 'Acute Compartmental Syndrome'. The first priority is to salvage the foot/limb by decompressing the compartment by doing fasciotomy. Once this is achieved, other treatments can follow.

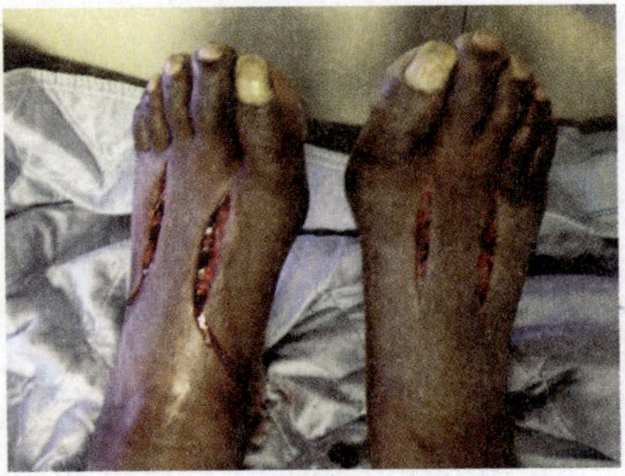

Fasciotomy

Q12: Meena, 50, is my colleague in office. She sustained a small fracture at the wrist after a fall from a two wheeler but even after the fracture union, surprisingly, her fingers, elbow and shoulder are painfully stiff. Why?

Although Meena had a small fracture in the wrist which may have united in a month's time, the painful stiffness in the fingers, elbow and shoulder of that particular limb is due to a syndrome called 'Reflex Sympathetic Dystrophy' which can affect non injured areas of the limb too. This is an unfortunate development in some patients which happens due to exaggerated response to the pain. Certain chemicals are secreted and they lead to pain and stiffness in the whole limb. The worst part of the story is, it is a self-limiting disease which usually takes upto one year for improvement and no medicine can cure it instantly. Physiotherapy and supportive treatment does help.

Q13: How to bring an amputated limb or hand to the hospital?

After a wash to get rid of dust and dirt, very quickly it should be put in a clean polybag and that bag should be further put into a large polybag with lots of ice. This will keep the amputated part cool but not directly in contact with ice. Usually, the safe time for re-implantation surgeries in such cases is six hours. But some surgeons have tried it successfully even later. Advisory in such an emergency situation is to approach a higher care centre with quick response systems.

Q14: What do I do for ankle sprain?

RICE therapy is the answer—Rest, Ice packs, Compression and Elevation. In case, injury doesn't settle in 3-4 days, it's better to get a below knee plaster done by orthopedic surgeon for a period of 3 to 6 weeks. The duration of plaster cast is generally decided by severity of injury and clinical assessment by orthopedic surgeons.

Nowadays, instead of old-fashioned white Plaster of Paris, fiber cast is applied which is light and strong; allows easy walk and routine activity.

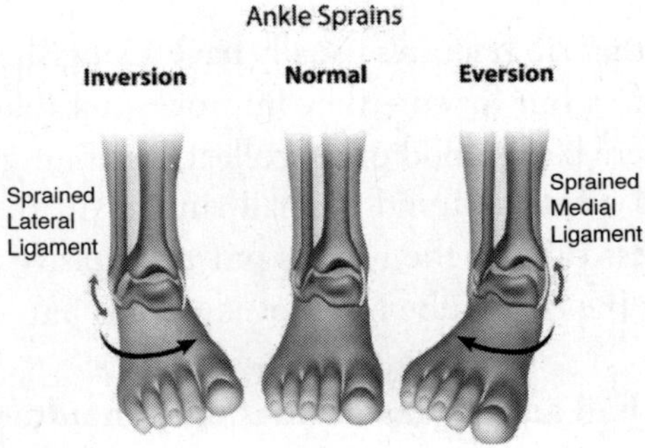

Q15: It was a horrible experience for my friend to have fractured three ribs in chest but the orthopedic took it so lightly, no plaster—nothing?

Blunt injury to the chest might have resulted in fracture of 3 ribs on one side of chest, which is an extremely painful situation, especially during breathing, coughing or sneezing. Although pain is excruciating, unfortunately, no POP plaster is done on chest for immobilisation.

The only thing done is rib binder application (something like bolt) in full expiration which partially reduces ribcage movements and reduces pain. Yes, the X-ray has to be properly looked at for any haemothorax (blood collection in lungs) or pneumothorax (air collection in lungs) which can cause respiratory problem and in such cases, patient should be admitted in a hospital.

It looks like, your friend had just 3 rib fractures which will heal in 4-6 weeks and was therefore treated in OPD and sent home.

I agree that rib fractures usually have a longish spell of discomfort but for sure they improve after that.
Had there been blood or air collection in lungs, then hospital admission and a small surgery in the form of a chest tube in the lung is put to improve affairs. Usually the chest tube is removed within 3 to 4 days.

Q16: I had an impression that only shoulder joint dislocates, but was greatly horrified to hear that following a fall from a bike, my friend had an elbow dislocated. Will he be back to normal ever?

Elbow dislocation is not as common as shoulder dislocation but it does happen. Your friend's elbow must have been properly relocated to normal position and immobilised for 1 month (to avoid recurrence) by an orthopedic at hospital. After 1 month he will need good amount of exercises to gain normal movements but ultimately the elbow will be functional.
Sometimes the dislocation may be associated with fracture around elbow and in that case the situation can be all the more tricky. A CT scan analysis and proper non-operative or operative treatment needs to be done.

Q17: My aunt had a knee dislocation which was set by an ortho specialist, but she can't lift her foot even after 4 months. What to do?

Knee dislocation is a very serious injury and usually happens with high intensity trauma. The leg bone and thigh bone face each other and work in synchrony. When your aunt had a dislocation, the leg bone went backwards and pressed on blood vessels and there is stretching of the common perennial nerve on outer side of knee, which is responsible for lifting of foot. In her case, post reduction of knee by the doctor, the vessels have not suffered any damage (in some cases there can be loss of blood supply to leg also), but the nerve has suffered a damage leading to foot-drop. Now she can't lift foot upwards and it is called 'high gait'. She may recover in 1-year period automatically with the help of some medicinal support. In case it doesn't, surgery to transfer tendon for lifting foot can be done.

Your aunt can undergo Nerve Conduction Velocity (NCV) test and EMG (Electromyography) test and know the recovery status of the nerve. I agree that because of prolonged recovery phase, the patient can be impatient at times.

Q18: My young cousin underwent surgery for fractured thigh bone. Post operatively on the 2nd day of operation, he went breathless and later collapsed? Is it the doctor's negligence?

It is a very unfortunate complication of fracture which is called fat embolism (where bone marrow fat dislodges and lodges in lungs). It can happen before or after surgery. It is bad luck of the surgeon also, though a low molecular weight heparin (clot dissolving medicines) can prevent and treat the problem, there is no guarantee about prevention and success of treatment. No doubt it is a huge loss, but any medico-legal case against the doctor will be unfair.

Q19: My grandmother was operated for hip fracture by an orthopedic surgeon at a big hospital. The fracture has not united. Should I go to court?

Well, you are free to approach the court but non-union of a fracture in your grandmother's body is not a doctor's making. She is old and the union depends on the type of the fracture too. There can be many reasons for her nonunion, you have to discuss with your surgeon and find best solution to ameliorate her suffering.

Q20: My brother's fracture in the leg bone didn't unite in plaster for 4 months. Later our orthopedic surgeon operated on his leg, with plating and bone grafting. Now the leg is 2cm short. Can we get compensation from a consumer court?

It depends on the counseling to patient and attendants. It is but natural that in a nonunion tibia (leg bone), some refreshing of fractured ends is required and then fixation is done. Bone graft is to promote union. Refreshing and sacrificing edges at fracture ends will lead to shortening but in case your doctor has not taken you in confidence about this fallout, you may approach consumer court for compensation. Medico legal issue apart, upto 1 cm shortening in leg is hardly of any consequence.

In this case poor communication and absence of informed consent is the main issue and definitely there is no medical negligence.

Q21a: After a neck (cervical) fracture in a road accident my maternal uncle got completely paralysed. Does he have any chance?

In cervical spine injury, if the vertebra (bone) has gone backwards to press on the spinal cord, then post decompression and fixation surgery recovery is good. But, when the spinal cord is transacted or irreparably damaged, Quadriplegia (paralysis of all 4 limbs) or paraplegia (paralysis of two lower limb) or monoplegia (paralysis of one limb) would be the outcome. This is what has happened to your uncle. Complete transaction has no cure, only nursing care is the answer.

Physiotherapy, occupational therapy and bladder/ bowel training is very important for rehabilitation of such patients. See to it, he does not develop bedsores.

Q21b: Can he die because of bedsore?

Yes, many a time when a patient is diabetic or immune-compromised, he can go into septicemic shock and may die. Total surveillance is required for such cases.

Q21c.: My uncle has also developed deep bedsore despite so much care, what is the remedy?

If your uncle is having superficial bedsore then daily dressing, sitting and turning in bed half hourly, facilitates healing in a few days. Don't lose patience and perseverance.

If the bedsore is deep, then pus culture and sensitivity, antibiotics, dressings are the minimum treatment. At times, it needs surgery by a plastic surgeon. It is a challenge to handle deep bedsores and the best is to prevent such an eventuality.

Sports Injuries

Q1: Being a sports loving boy, I play field games regularly. How to avoid and take care of injuries?

The best way is to have a 15-minute warm up and gentle exercises before actual play. Drink water in between the game to avoid dehydration. Stretching exercises of upper and lower body are important for good body balance. Above all, know your limits; an athlete or player is advised to push him or herself not beyond 10 to 15% of the known capacity or performance in a particular game/event.

Q2: My cousin is a kabaddi player, having very good muscles. But his shoulder has been dislocated 4 times in the past one year. What is the trouble?

Shoulder joint is a highly mobile joint with a big ball (round head of upper arm bone, Humerus) sitting on a small saucer shaped surface (1/8th diameter of head) of a triangular wing-like bone called 'scapula' on which the arm rotates almost 360⁰. An additional depth to this articulation of ball and socket is provided by ligaments and brim of hard tissue called labrum. Any defect in the brim or wall of labrum or tear in the capsule due to forceful movements can bring the top ball of arm bone out of the socket. This is called 'dislocation' which is very painful and a critical situation.

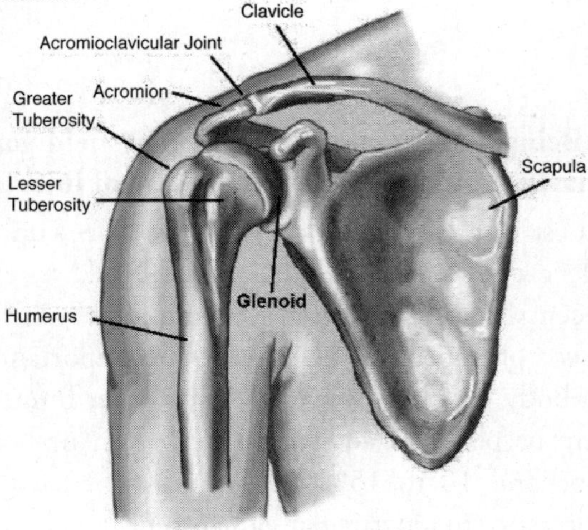

Once the orthopedist reduces the joint by manipulation, it is mandatory to immobilise the shoulder for 1 month by shoulder immobiliser despite no complaint of pain. Many a time, the patient takes this advice very casually and starts working, which in turn impedes complete healing of the torn labrum and capsule. Such cases usually have recurrence of dislocation in certain rotatory movements of shoulder.

Your cousin also appears to be having this problem. Although it is easy to reduce (set) the shoulder back to socket every time, but a permanent solution is surgery which is through open or arthroscopic (key-hole) access. There are some surgeries described and performed mostly on the soft tissue and the muscle repair with some restriction of external rotation of arm, having almost 85-90% success rate. No surgery is 100% fool proof.

Q3: Although throwing stones is a simple act, my son is unable to do it after a small sports injury. What can it be?

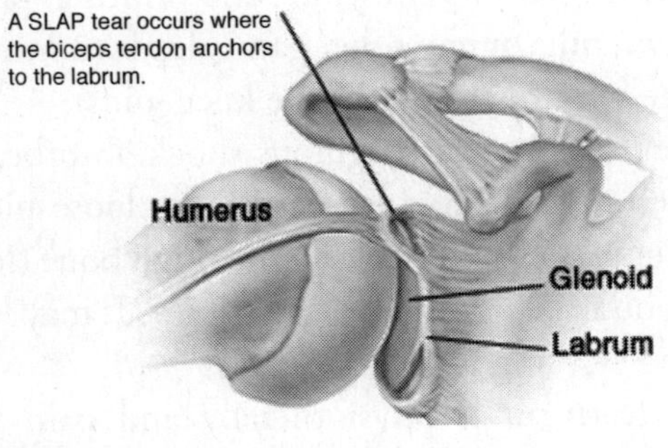

Most likely it is a SLAP tear (Superior Labrum Anterior Posterior). It is a tear in the cartilaginous boundary wall of the Glenoid (saucer like socket of shoulder). There can be mild to severe grades of tear. It usually happens either due to a fall or injury on outstretched hand or vigorous overhead playing activity.

Besides pain and instability, there will be difficulty in throwing the stone/ball. This needs pain killers and physiotherapy as initial treatment and if it doesn't settle, arthroscopic surgery is the answer, where anchors (small screws) are put to reattach the labrum boundary to the Glenoid bony saucer tightly. This is followed by a 3-weeks rest in arm pouch, followed by good exercises and rehabilitation programme for ten weeks. The results are good.

Q4: My knee was injured during a tennis game and it locks during movements although the pain is not unbearable. Is it serious?

The twisting injury in your knee during playing, whether tennis or any other game, leads to miniscule tear (the semilunar bush in the knee joint).

The meniscus is a cartilaginous shock absorber kind of structure and gets torn easily; the loose piece of meniscus gets caught between the thigh bone (femur) and leg bone (tibia) and locks the joint. It may lead to pain and swelling too.

Initial treatment is physiotherapy and pain killers for at least 2 weeks. If it doesn't work, then key hole surgery (arthroscopy) of knee is done. The option is of excising the torn part, smoothening the edges and in some cases, repair of the tear.

Usually results are good but in cases of complete meniscus removal, early onset of degenerative arthritis is the natural corollary.

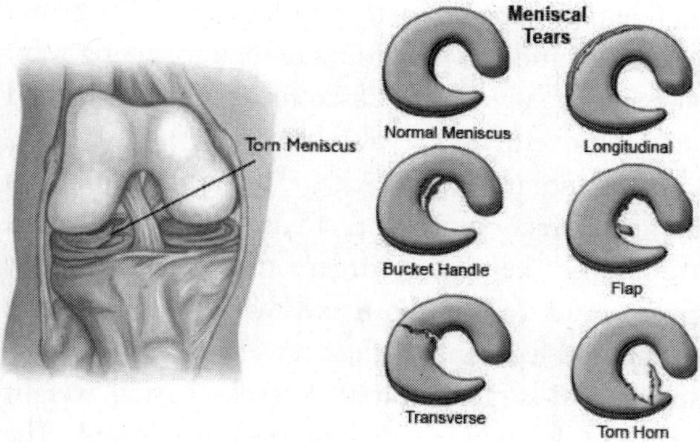

Q5: It was my brother's marriage party and during an over enthusiastic dance I fell down badly. There was no fracture but even after 2 months there is a feeling of laxity and giving way of knee. What can it be?

Apparently, in your case it looks like an anterior cruciate ligament tear (ACL).The rope like structure is the one which attaches and binds leg bone (Tibia) with the thigh bone (Femur).

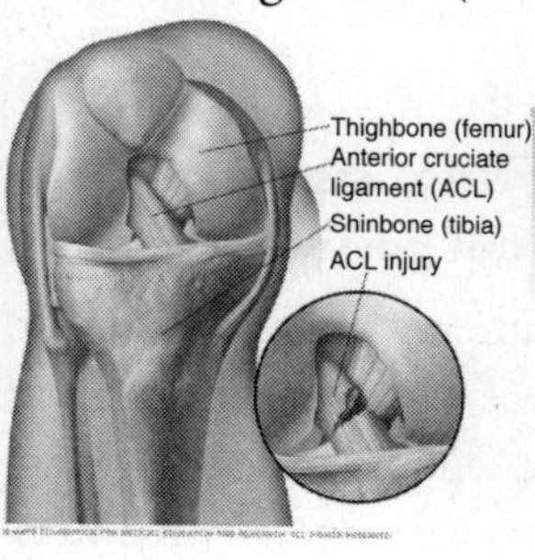

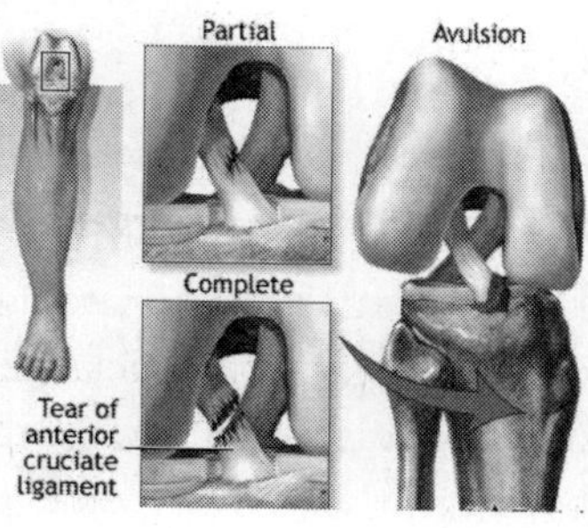

The ligaments are important to keep joints together while laxity and forward going tendency (giving way) makes joint unstable. Discomfort and disturbed range of movements can also be there.

As a temporary relief ice, elevation, painkillers and knee brace support is advised but finally the arthroscopic (key hole) surgery to recreate the new ligament and tie it on both ends with two bio screws in thigh and leg bones is the answer.

Usually post-surgery, initial 3 weeks partial weight bearing walk with crutches or stick is allowed. The normal life is resumed at 6 weeks but driving bike is permitted at 3 months and athletic activity can begin after 6 months of surgery.

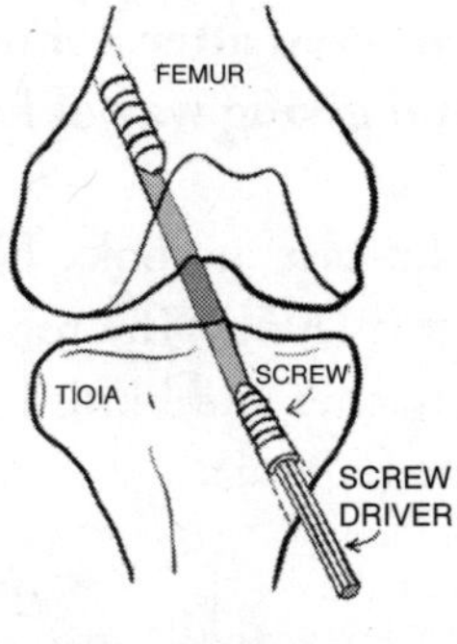

Q6: What is the trouble if knee sags backwards and running and jogging is not possible?

Like the anterior cruciate ligament, there is posterior cruciate ligament (backside of knee), again a rope like structure. If it breaks, the leg bone starts sagging backwards and can't take pressure. It also requires reconstruction. These ligaments do not grow and repair on their own like bone and skin due to poor blood supply.

Normally the tendons (white muscle belly extensions) on internal side of knee—called hamstring tendons—are harvested and are used for reconstruction of anterior and posterior cruciate ligaments. The tendons are dispensable and removal from original place doesn't create any deficiency in a limb.

Such injuries are common sports injuries, although treatment is possible and results are gratifying but recovery curve is slow and before a professional player can reach the same level of activity, it may be six months to one year.

Q7: While playing badminton last week I had a twisting sprain of my right wrist. Despite one week off from the game it is not improving, why?

Yes, you are rightly experiencing this nagging pain which is mostly at the inner side of wrist (the little finger side) due to partial tear of ulnar collateral ligament. This pain can be felt most at the tip of the bone and usually doesn't settle down with ice and pain killers (the first line of treatment). It is wise to go for one month of below elbow plaster, POP or fiber cast, which provides complete rest. Immobilisation provides healing environment and it is the best solution in the long run.

Shoulder Elbow Wrist Hand

Q1: My father is diabetic and recently had angioplasty also. After that he is not able to move his shoulders freely at all. What to do?

This is a condition called frozen shoulder where all the movements of shoulder are restricted and painful. Shoulder may be painful during the rest period also, say at night. Pain may refer to arm in many patients. In your father's case, the diabetes has led to adhesive capsulitis, ie. the joint capsule is contracted and is not allowing the bones to move freely; trigger being reduced activity of shoulder after angioplasty. For that matter, any procedure like bypass heart surgery when shoulders are not actively used, may precipitate the disease.

The solution is simple exercises of shoulders and ultrasonic therapy at physiotherapy center can be taken up for a few weeks. Control the sugar, take simple pain killers. If situation is not improving, the orthopedic can inject local steroids into the joint. But before giving this shot, ascertain that blood sugar level is normal to avoid infection.

Q2: I am a woman of 52 years and I do not suffer from any disease. I just fell down on my shoulder and the X-Ray shows no bony injury. Yet, I can't lift my shoulder for the last 3 weeks? Why?

Usually in such cases, when there is no bony injury, the shoulder remains painful for some weeks and local tenderness of the shoulder joint would occur due to Supraspinatus tendinitis, which means the muscle Supraspinatus (responsible for lifting the shoulder) is torn partially or completely. In cases of partial tear, physiotherapy and pain killers will improve the situation but if the tendon looks completely

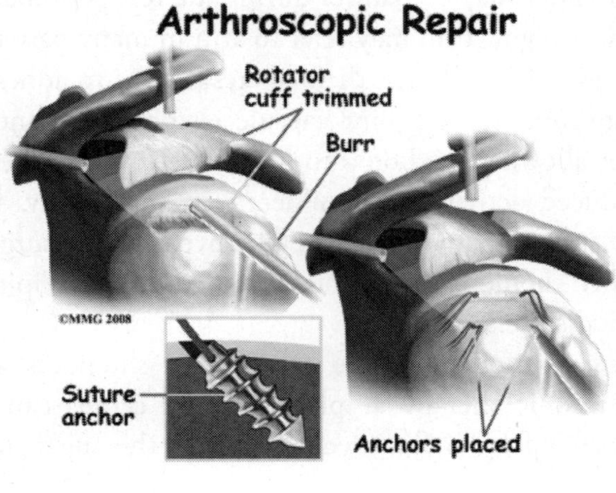

torn and there is no improvement, go for an MRI confirmation. Once confirmed, Arthroscopic surgery (key-hole surgery) can be performed to repair the tear using special anchors. Patients usually improves within six weeks.

Q3: My wife cannot lift a pressure cooker in the kitchen or wash clothes due to pain in the right elbow. Even while she is at rest, there is slight discomfort on the outer side of the elbow. What is the problem?

Your wife is probably suffering from an ailment called 'Tennis Elbow'. All the muscles at the back of the forearm which are responsible for extension of fingers and wrist are attached to the bone on the outer side of the elbow, ie. the lower end of the upper arm bone called 'Humerus' swelling due to stretching or weight lifting is a common symptom at this site. There is a similar condition called 'Golfers Elbow Fexor Tenosynovitis (swelling around tendon insertion)' on inner side of elbow. In golfers' elbow, the muscle group involved in the activity are in the front of the forearm.

Treatment of choice: giving rest to the elbow, avoid lifting weight, analgesics like paracetamol NSAIDs and applying moist heat for some days. In more severe cases local injection of a steroid is advised by an orthopedist (1 or 2 times would be sufficient) in addition to the physiotherapy, like ultrasonic therapy.

Q4: My thumb straightens with a snap like a knife and is paining for almost past two months. I am frustrated despite the use of pain killers. Is there any chance of improvement?

Medically the ailment is 'Stenosing Flexor Tenosynovitis' or 'Trigger thumb'. Such constricting tightness of tendon sheath which bends the thumb can also happen in other fingers. The problem can be precipitated due to specific tasks like writing, driving, computer typing, playing musical instruments and cooking. It may also be associated with diabetes and underlying joint diseases like Rheumatoid arthritis, connective tissue disorders and hypothyroidism. This association needs to be ruled out. Ailment of minor degree can be cured with hot water fomentation, exercises and analgesics but if it doesn't improve, local steroid in the tendon sheath of thumb is given by an orthopedist (usually single shot is sufficient). In about 15% cases, the condition is severe and need Tendon release surgery which means the sheath of Flexor tendon is cut and the tendon is released. Results are good and instant.

Q5: What does a hot painful shoulder mean in a child? Is the discomfort treatable? It happened to my maid's 10-year-old son and the doctors painted a very gloomy picture. Can you elaborate?

This looks like a purulent acute infection of shoulder joint, where the joint is most likely having pus.

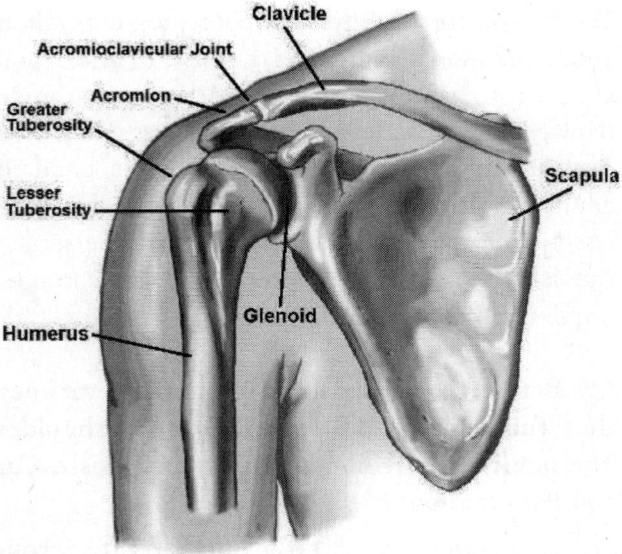

Usually such infections spread through blood (hematogenous), with source being elsewhere like throat, urinary tract or boil on the skin.

Sometimes, when the infection is not very virulent and is identified at the early stage, intravenous antibiotics can cure it, with the results visible within 48-72 hours. But, in case the pus is evident and blood investigations (in form of high leucocyte/neutrophil count) are supporting the diagnosis, the best option is the surgery called arthrotomy. In this, after opening the joint, all pus and dead tissue are debrided and washed out of the joint. After surgery, the patient is advised to take antibiotics for a few weeks, initially as intravenous and later by the oral route.

Yes, the doctors rightly said 'poor prognosis' about your maid's son because after the onset of infection in children, the growing plate called Epiphysis can get damaged. This can lead to gross stiffness and growth disturbance of upper limb too. Unlike children, adults (18+) have fused Epiphysis, so the damage is less but nevertheless, stiffness following the surgery can happen. This usually improves with sustained physiotherapy (exercises).

Q6: Before it happened to my old aunt, I never knew that Tuberculosis (TB) can happen in shoulder. The family is horrified about the prognosis. Can you tell me about it?

The commonest site of TB is lungs and the second commonest is the musculoskeletal system. TB in shoulder, although not very common, is a definite entity and needs proper treatment.

Chronic pain, warmth, restriction of movements, wasting of muscles and swelling which is not settling with pain killers and even with antibiotics; one should rule out TB of shoulder. X ray, blood investigation and/or an MRI can clinch the diagnosis.

Initial treatment is usually the anti TB drugs. Four- to 5-drug therapy for 3 months, then 3 drugs up to 6 months and 2 drugs upto one-and-a-half years is the usual regime. The shoulder arm immobiliser is used for first 6 weeks to provide rest to part. The results start showing in 6 weeks time. In intractable cases where blood investigations and clinical findings show no improvement for 8 weeks, surgical intervention in the form of open or arthroscopic surgery is done. Usually joint wash (lavage), synovial Biopsy (small piece of the grease forming membrane around joints taken out) and/or the joint fluid for special TB (AFB) culture and sensitivity can be done. All this will help in identifying and treating the TB in a much better way. Usually conservative treatment is sufficient and disease settles down in a period of one-and-a-half years.

Q7: My wife has a round swelling of a coin size at the back of her wrist which she ignored earlier, until it turned painful. Is it a tumour? Is there anything to worry?

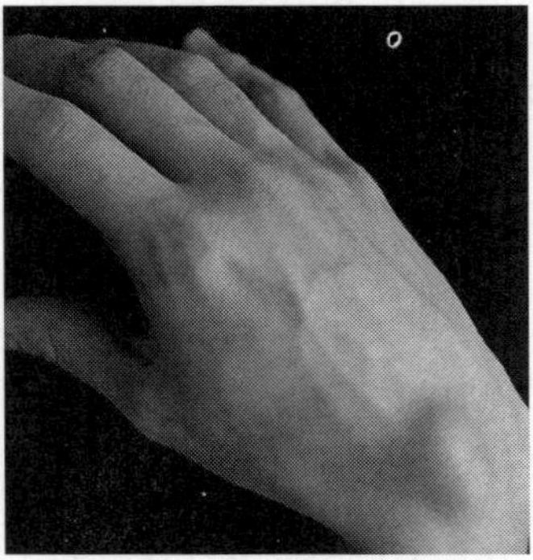

Counsel your wife not to worry. Such a swelling at the back of the wrist is most likely benign in nature (not cancerous), in medical parlance it is called Ganglion. The ganglion is mobile and originates from the tendon or joint capsule. In the initial stages, it is painless but later due to degeneration or pressure on some nerve in the vicinity it can become painful. The conservative line of treatment is aspiration of the content (jelly like) from the ganglion and pushing an injectable steroid in it. It usually settles down. But, in case it doesn't, then surgical excision and biopsy is done. The originating base is usually cauterised to prevent recurrence. Nevertheless, no guarantee can be furnished about its recurrence.

Q8: My senior colleague in office developed a strange problem. His ring and little finger were drawn towards palm and he can't straighten them. What can it be?

For reasons not fully known, some people, mostly in old age especially, develop a condition of fibrotic changes in the fascia underneath the skin of palm (from wrist to fingers). The ailment is called Duputran's contracture, in which, the palmer fascia develops cord like strands and in severe cases the fingers can even dig into the palm. Probably your senior colleague has this ailment.

In the initial stages multiple needling in the facial cord releases the tightness and should be followed by physiotherapy. In later stages, a surgery to release the cords would be needed. Apparently this condition is less prevalent in India and more in western countries.

Q9: My wife has been complaining of pain in the right wrist along with numbness in right thumb and index finger. Despite lots of medication nothing is improving. Why?

It seems that your wife is suffering from a condition called 'Carpal Tunnel Syndrome'. In this condition, a nerve (called median nerve) gets compressed usually without any trauma at the palmer side of the wrist. The compression of nerve leads to weakness in the pinch, numbness of thumb, index finger and middle finger and adjoining area. Diagnosis can be confirmed by nerve conduction test costing about two-three thousand rupees and once confirmed, the nerve can be surgically decompressed. It's a small surgery with gratifying results.

Q10: My mother, 50 years old, has been suffering from Tendinitis of rotator cuff shoulder for the last one year. We have tried all treatments and nothing works. Are there any advanced treatments for this?

No doubt, tendinitis of rotator cuff shoulder, tennis elbow, planter fasciitis are certain very intractable situations to treat and patients don't improve despite physiotherapy, local steroids medicines, rest etc.

The latest advanced therapy of plasma extract is a new treatment. This is an OPD procedure, whereby patient's own blood is taken out (5 ml), centrifuged in machine and plasma is separated and injected (cells

are removed completely) at the affected site.
There are two issues, one, it costs Rs 15,000 to 20,000. Two, effectivity is still doubtful.

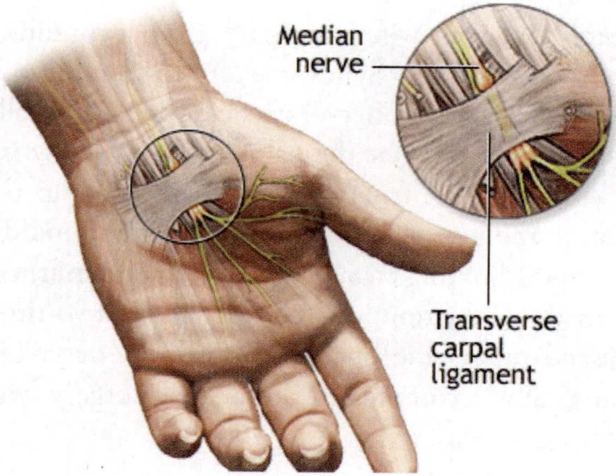

Neck and Back

Q1: My grandfather always keeps complaining of neck pain and stiffness and now my father, who is just 55, is also going the same way. What should I do for them and also to save myself?

Yes, neck pains in elderly people like your grandpa and father is most likely due to degenerative changes in cervical (neck area) spine. The ailment is called cervical spondylitis. The spine from head to tailbone has 28 bones, out of it 7 are in neck and as the neck has too much of movement like bending forward, extending, rotating to sides, damages are earlier in this part of the spine than in the dorsal spine (the area behind chest).

There is indeed a 'lifestyle' dimension to it and also another important dimension is genetic. But unfortunately, you can't do much for genetic risk but you can very well have a lifestyle which is good for the neck. Avoid bending of neck forward while reading or cooking, this is advisory for all age groups. Besides pain killers and muscle relaxants for a short period, local applications of painkilling gel and hot water bag helps. Elevating the desk or computer keyboard/ laptop for easy working is good for teachers, office executives, penpushers, students, software engineers, accountants, lawyers and even for family physicians who keep writing prescriptions seven to eight hours a day.

For your grandpa, formal physiotherapy sessions with exercises and machines will be a good idea for 10-15 days in crisis state. Later he can do 10-15 mins exercise twice daily at home

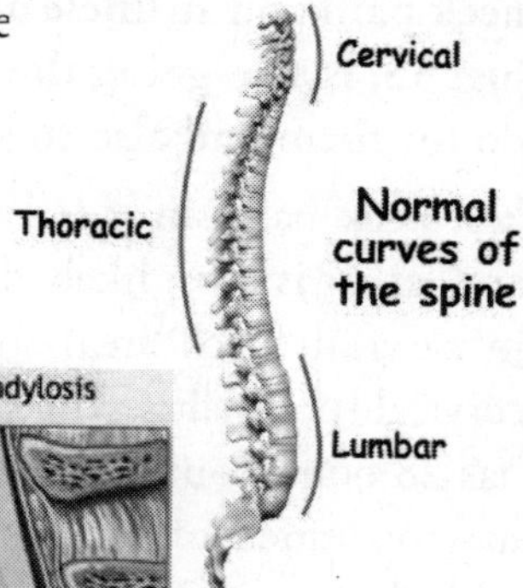

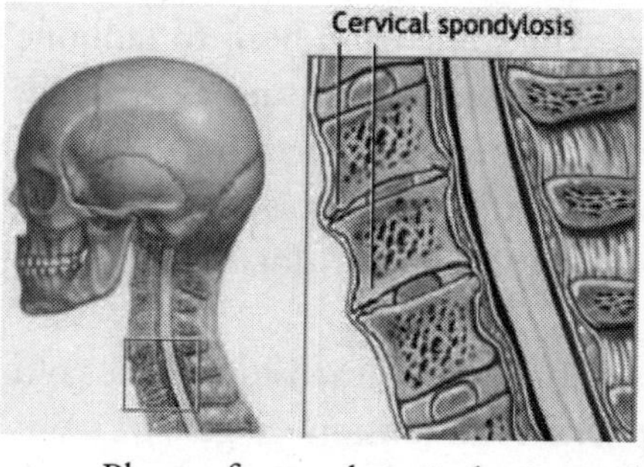

Photo of normal cervical spine and degenerated spine side by side

Q2: Whenever somebody gets pain in the neck, colleagues say, this is cervical; what exactly is it? I had an impression that only elderly people have this ailment.

First of all 'Cervical' is not a disease, it is actually the part of the spine corresponding to the neck and it has seven small squarish bones called cervical vertebrae. The whole spine from head to hips has 28 such bones and joints on sides for interconnection.

Now, the problem of your office colleagues who have sitting jobs of 5 to 8 hours every day, be it on computer or file work, the constant forward bending of neck leads to pain and stiffness. The muscles and ligaments get taught and go into spasm and these friends will constantly complain of neck problem. They need to mount keyboards and screens at elevated heights so that there is no bending of neck. Also, after every one hour, they should take a break of 10 minutes, relax the neck shoulder muscles (gentle exercises), stroll around and then again settle down to desk work.

There are studies to indicate that such people also have early cervical spondylitis or may be it precipitates because of their not-so-neck-friendly life style.

Beyond the office also, all such sedentary workers should perform stretching exercises of the whole body, go for walk or jogging or get involved in some field game for at least 45 minutes daily. Specifically, 10 minutes daily devoted to neck exercises will help in a big way. So, this advisory is important for software engineers, charted accountants, teachers, clerical staff, shopkeepers (sitting at cash counters) and receptionists.

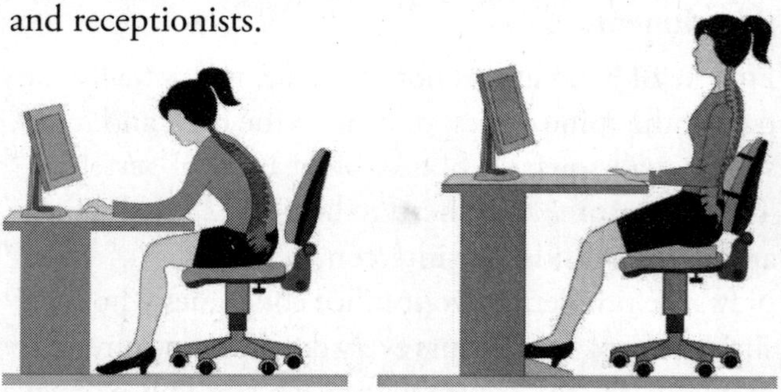

Q3: I am a designer of 28 years and suffer from on/off low backache. When I was assessed, nothing positive came out. Similar is the issue with my IT field friends too. How to be fully fit?

Don't worry, you are not alone. There are millions of people who are suffering from low backache. In fact, low backache is so common that many ortho centers run special low backache clinics. And, as you said, after all investigations like blood, X-ray and MRI nothing positive came out. It only shows there is no serious disease per say but something wrong for sure. IT professionals, computer operators and all those who have long sitting hours develop weak muscles, stiffness in paraspinal muscles (adjoining the spine) and ligaments; you may say this is an occupational hazard but there are ways to fight it.

Change lifestyle—avoid sitting for more than 1 hour at a time. Get up on hourly basis to relax your muscles and sit again after 10 minutes. Learn the extension exercises of back from physiotherapist for seven days and then keep doing those exercises daily for at least 15 minutes to strengthen your back. Just try this and you will experience thrilling results.

Quite likely that people above 45-50 may already have early or moderate changes of lumbar spondylitis (degenerative changes in lower 5 lumbar vertebra) which can be the reason for pain and stiffness. More so in the early morning. The uneven bony edges and growths of vertebra in spondylitis can impinge

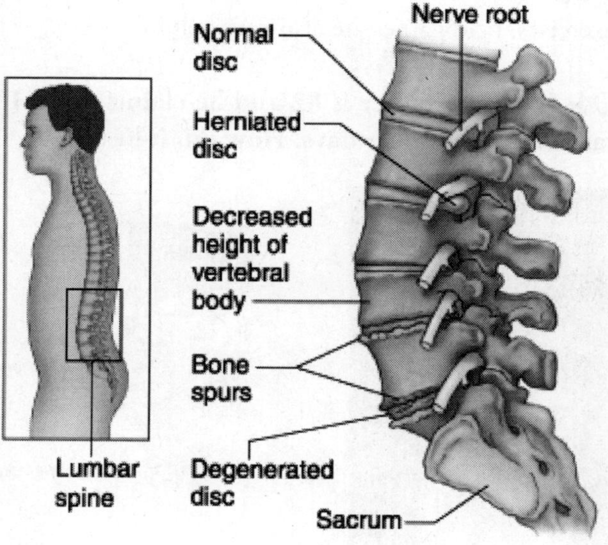

on muscles and sometimes on nerves, which can produce spasm of muscles and radiation of pain to legs consecutively. Also, the disc (a spongy cushion) between the rectangular vertebras may also degenerate in later stages. Once the disc collapses, the facet joints (intervertebral side joints) come under stress, leading to further pain.

The solution is to adopt correct sitting posture, sleeping in lateral position, muscle relaxants, nerve energisers and repairing drugs, pain killers, back support belts, local applications of pain relieving creams and above all, physiotherapy (exercises of back with temporary use of gadgets like diathermy, IFT etc). A general active lifestyle in form of walk, jogging, stretching exercises, field games are also very helpful.

Q4: My grandfather is 82 and he claims to be 1" taller in his younger days. How can it be so?

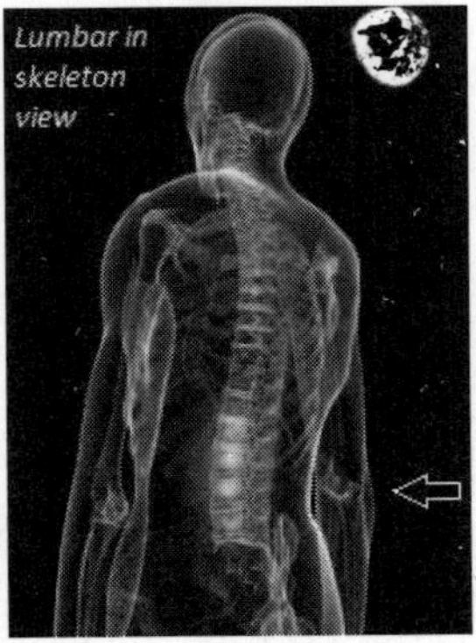

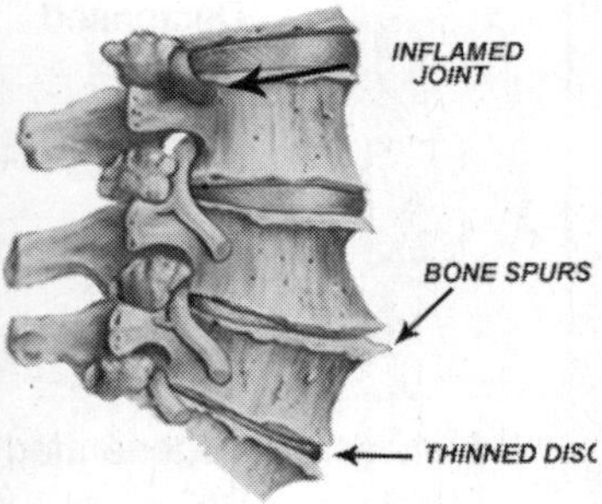

Yes, he is right. With advancing age, the intervertebral discs (spongy rubber cushion between the rectangular vertebrae of spine) lose their moisture and height. Naturally, the reduced height of spine is cause for reduction in height in old age. This may be up to 1 inch. Also apparently due to stiffness of neck and back, the very elderly tend to walk with a little bent posture. Usually all this is a very gradual degeneration and doesn't require any special treatment except some physiotherapy.

Q5: At railway stations, the coolies keep lifting bags for years but nothing happens; I lifted a large flower pot in my garden and doctor says it is a big disc prolapse. Needs surgery. Strange?

Your argument looks genuine at face value. But in medicine it is not 2+2=4. The coolie may or may not have disc prolapse but these are two different cases.

Usually, in acute disc prolapse, conservative treatment in the form of rest, pain killers and physiotherapy is good enough. Rest may go on from 1 week to 4 weeks. In small percentage of severe cases, the MRI confirms complete herniation of disc material which sits on spinal cord at the backside or compresses nerve significantly. Then surgery is indicated in the form of decompression, discectomy with or without microscope. Normally, surgery is an option for chronic cases, recurrent cases and those who do not improve with conservative treatment.

Nowadays, if surgery of 2-level disc decompression is done, then pedicle screws with rods are also used for fixation from backside. This provides additional strength to spine. But many surgeons are of the opinion that fixation is not required in routine cases.

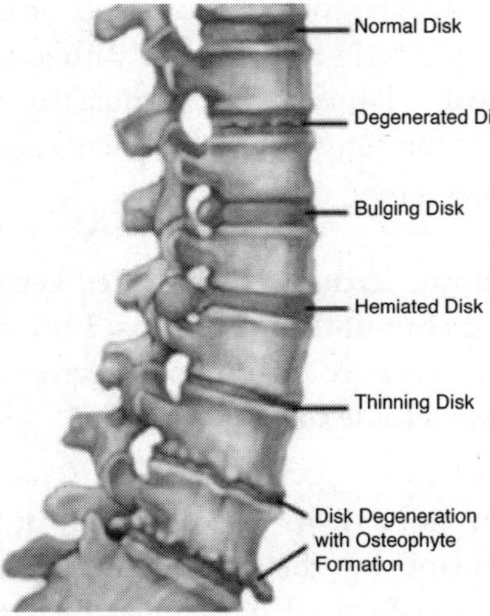

Q6a: My husband was having backache for the last three months. The doctor has declared after assessment that it is TB of spine. How to be sure and can it affect other members of family?

I am sure your husband must be having positive blood indicators and positive findings in MRI; after corroborating these with clinical picture, the doctor would have labeled him as TB spine. More proof usually is not required but in case of any doubt, a

histopathology (biopsy) test from the diseased vertebra of the spine by thick needle under CT scan guidance can be conclusive.
There is nothing to worry as bone TB is not contagious; TB spreads only from lungs (sputum/cough).

Q6b: I am extremely worried for my husband, people told me TB of spine leads to paralysis. Is it so?

Yes. TB of spine, if not treated properly, can lead to paralysis of upper and/or lower limbs, depending on the level of involvement in the spine. Like TB of cervical spine (neck) may result in paralysis of all four limbs while that of dorso-lumbar spine (back) will only give rise to lower limbs paralysis.

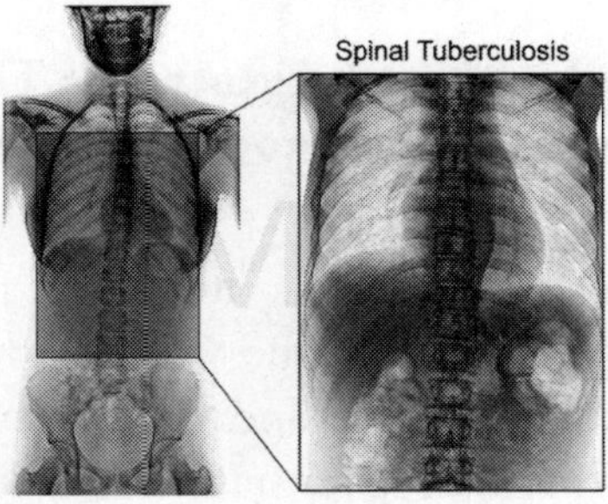

This is because the pus, disease material (granulation tissue) and collapsed bone vertebra press the spinal cord from behind. This results in loss of motor power in the body below this level of disease. Besides the mechanical pressure, the reduced blood supply and absorbed toxins can cause neurological deficiency (loss of strength and sensation).

Q6c: The doctor has prescribed rest and anti TB drugs to my husband, will it be enough for cure?

Normally anti TB drugs, complete rest and minimal movement limited to toilet going, with spine support brace are advised. Usually, within 6 weeks, progress should be visible and also assessed through blood investigations and MRI. If there is no improvement even after 2 months and there is a deterioration, it may turn out to be the case of multi drug resistant TB, which is more dangerous and needs more evaluation and different set of drugs.

Alertness is important in spine TB, otherwise paraplegia (loss of power in limbs) will follow sooner or later.

Q6d: I have heard second generation TB drugs are very expensive and have too many side effects, is it true?

Yes, it is true. But there is no reason to push the panic button, a step in time will go a long way in controlling the TB spine and your husband can be normal. The multi drug resistant TB has less than 3% side effects.

Q6e: What will be the duration of my husband's therapy?

Cure of spine TB takes normally 18 months, which is double the time taken for cure of lung TB.

Q6f: Does he need any surgery?

Yes. If he is not improving and there are chances of imminent paralysis or if the paralysis of limbs with or without urine and bowel involvement is already there, surgery is the only option. Surgery means cleaning the pus, decompression of spinal cord and stabilisation of spine by pedicle screws and rods.

This surgery helps in control of disease focus, early mobilisation of patient and gives better results. If followed by full anti-TB drugs therapy, usually results are gratifying.

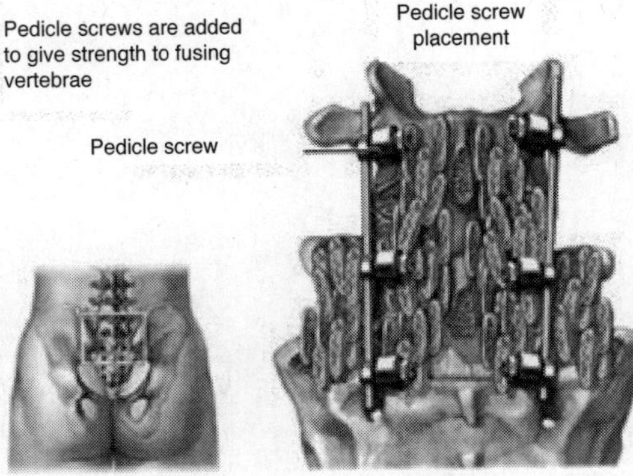

Q7: My Uncle's daughter is just 12 and has a very curvaceous and hunched spine. What is her future?

In a normally vertical spine, a curvature towards side is called Scoliosis. This generally doesn't have a cause and scoliosis is more common in adolescent girls. The majority of such patients require 3-6 monthly follow-up including clinical examination and spine X-rays. The treatment is bracing in skeletally-immature patients, with mild to moderate degree of scoliosis and surgery in skeletally-mature patients with severe deformity. A similar ailment is when the curvature goes backwards. It is called kyphosis and is also treated on similar lines.

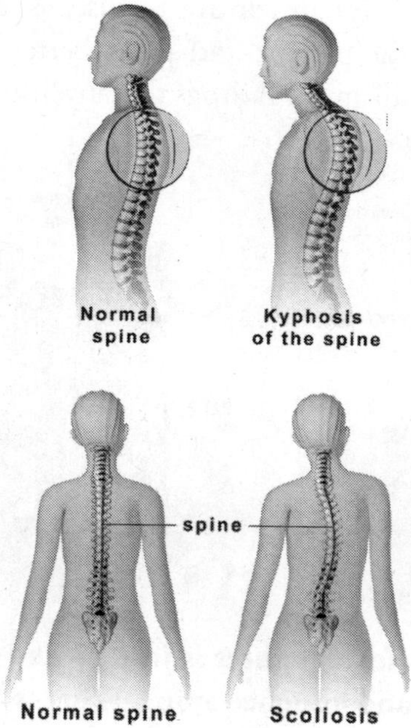

Arthritis

Q1: I am a teetotaler. I was under the impression that alcohol consumers may have gout but when our orthopaedician said that I have gout, I was greatly surprised.

Basic reason is disturbance in protein metabolism. Protein (purine) rich foods other than alcohol can cause gout and the urate crystals deposit in tendons, bursa and joints to cause pain and swelling, also the urate crystals can deposit in kidney to cause stones.

Q2: I am a marketing executive and travelling is an integral part of my job. Kindly advise as the recurrent pain at my right great toe bothers me too much.

Pain in the great toe or foot is most likely due to 'Gouty arthritis' or hyperuricemia(a type of joint disease). It most commonly affects foot/great toe but can also affect any other joint like knees, hands, back. In this disease the byproduct of protein metabolism, serum uric acid increases in blood and as a result deposits in joints, leading to pain and inflammation in joints. Normally a small blood test is good enough to ascertain that Serum uric acid level is below or above the normal value of 6 (the normal value may differ in different kits).

In case of a marketing executive like you who keeps on travelling, there are all the ingredients of mismanaged uric acid levels. Avoid high protein diet like grams (chana), kidney beans (rajma), white of eggs, tomato, brinjal, pulses, especially fish and meat. Secondly, alcohol and fructose-rich cold drinks are not advisable. Thirdly manage haphazard schedule and sleep deprivation.

If you can avoid all the above mentioned food items and other things, pain and swelling may settle down even without any medication and probably will not recur. Besides precautions, there are one or two medicines (uric acid lowering agents) which have to be temporarily taken for 1-2 weeks.

In some patients of hyperuricemia UAL agent needs to be continued for long duration too.

Q3: My mother is having bunion in foot, what to do for pain and deformity?

Bunion of great toe is mainly in people with wrong direction of foot bones. It is mainly due to weakness of ligament and joints. Wrong and tight footwear exacerbate the problem. Right footwear, silicon toe separator is helpful, bone correcting alignment surgery (osteotomy) is the final solution.

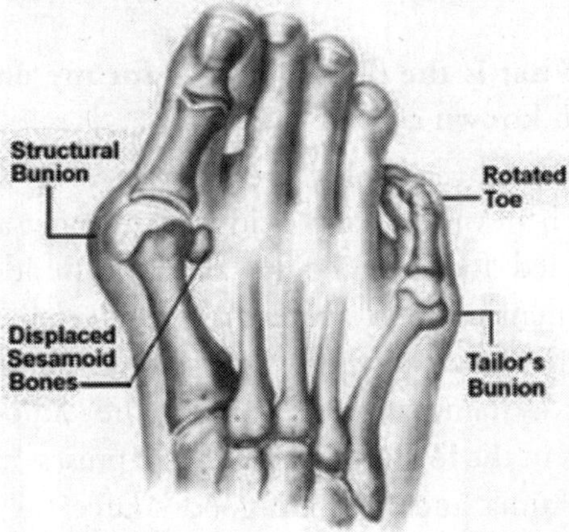

Q4a: My unmarried daughter, who is 25, has been diagnosed with rheumatoid arthritis recently, I am anxious about her future.

Well, rheumatoid arthritis (RA) is a joint disease in the young and usually a chronic disease controlled by medicines. If the RA factor is positive in blood (70%), usually it is a more severe type. The remaining 30% who are RA factor negative also suffer with multiple joint pains, but this is a relatively mild version.

As Your daughter is young, it calls for aggressive treatment with disease modifying drugs (DMARDS) on long term basis to take care of pain and prevent deformities. Yes the DMARDS therapy has some side effects on liver/kidney and blood, so needs to be monitored on regular basis.

With regular treatment, her future can be almost normal including her marital life.

Q4b: What is the dietary advice for my daughter who is a known case of RA?

Fresh fruits, vegetables, fresh water fish and sea food rich in omega fatty acids are strongly advised. Deep fried food should be avoided. Besides this, requirement of anti-oxidants is important which may be derived from citrus fruits oranges, gooseberry (Amla) (Vitamin C/A/E). Adequate amount of proteins in the forms of white of egg, pulses, chicken, grains, rajma and nuts are good source for muscle building and should always be consumed by your daughter.

Q5: My wife has Rheumatoid arthritis and has to be on NSAIDs (pain killers) and to beat that she takes daily antacids. Are antacids harmful?

Yes, long term use of antacids can be a cause of osteoporosis because it intervenes with the calcium absorption in gut. Therefore your wife needs to get her calcium, phosphorus and alkaline phosphatase checked in blood on yearly basis.

Also check her bone mineral density every 2 yearly, if less, then treat her for osteoporosis.

Q6: My friend, age 22 years, who was a known case of RA, had to undergo total hip replacement for both hips (Bilateral THR). As I am diagnosed with RA, should I go the same way?

Your friend is apparently a case of Juvenile RA that starts at an early age of 5 to 10 years and by the time one grows up to adulthood, in some cases, joints are destroyed. In such cases bilateral THR can be a possibility but you have been diagnosed with RA only in adulthood and definitely you will not travel exactly the same path. Still, In your case also, nobody can guarantee that joint will not be affected but with the new age medications, mostly it takes few decades and many a times, throughout life, a person may not need joint replacement. Stop worrying as proper treatment, exercises and diet will keep you healthy.

Q7: Unfortunately, my younger sister of 19 years, is a juvenile rheumatoid arthritis patient and her both hips require replacement. What kind of joint material will be most suitable for her?

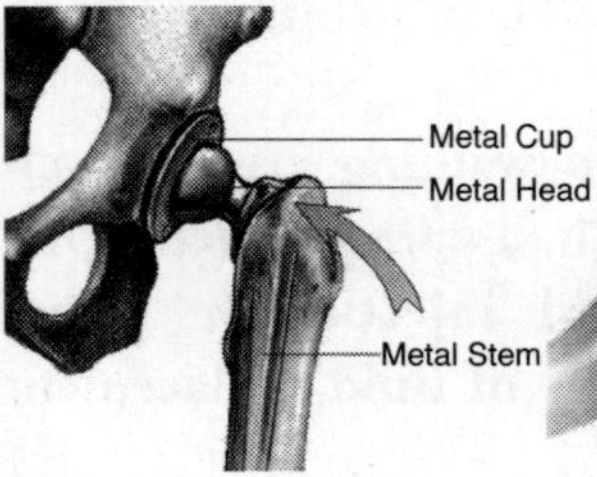

(Hip joint-METAL ON METAL)

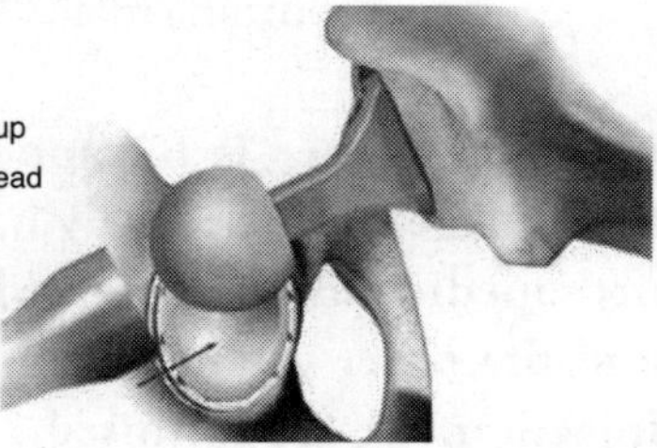

(Hip joint-Ceramic on Ceramic)

In her case metal on metal total hip joints (the roof acetabulum and head of thigh bone) is a bad idea. Young patients need uncemented hip for long life, either ceramic on polyethylene or oxinium on polyethylene or ceramic on ceramic hip bearing surfaces are good options.

Q8: I have read somewhere that Osteoarthritis (degenerative) type of joint arthritis happens to every second person above the age of 50, is it true? If yes, how can I save myself?

Yes, the incidence mentioned looks correct, although propensity is higher in women. Five factors have a big role and always remember them:

1. Keep weight under control.
2. Don't overlook knee limb deformities like knock knees or bow legs etc.
3. Don't ignore internal injuries of joints.
4. Early diagnosis and treatment helps, especially knees.
5. Hereditary predisposition (family history) has important role, so be watchful.

Q9: My mother is 82 and walking around well for her age. But she lately had pain in knees. One orthopedic advised steroid injection in joints and the other was in favour of fluid replacement injection. We are confused.

It is natural for you to be confused because as you say, at the age of 82 your mother is walking around well, that means degeneration (osteoarthritis) in her joints is not very bad and besides medicines and physiotherapy, intra-articular injection will benefit her.

Now let's talk about the two injections. Steroid shot is short term relief, may be for 1-2 months though it has some deleterious effect on joint cushion (called cartilage). Repeat injections definitely have. The synovial fluid therapy is a replacement of fluid naturally found in the knee. It has been bio engineered outside by companies and it has no side effects as such and it usually improves the knee for one year.

But the cost of steroid is Rs 200 while that of visco-supplementation is from 14 to 18 thousand rupees for an injection. When both ortho surgeons have advised injections, it is more a question of affordability and self-assessment.

find there are several different movements that make you dizzy, pick two to work on at a time. Once you no longer experience dizziness in response to these movements, add two more. Don't try to do exercises for more than two movements at a time.

Following are the common exercises which can be done. You can take a therapist's guidance initially if you wish:

Eye exercises

- Look up and down 20 times. Start slowly at first, then speed up.
- Look from one side to the other 20 times. Start slowly at first, then speed up.
- Hold up one finger at arm's length. Focus on it. Move it slowly in towards you and out again 20 times.

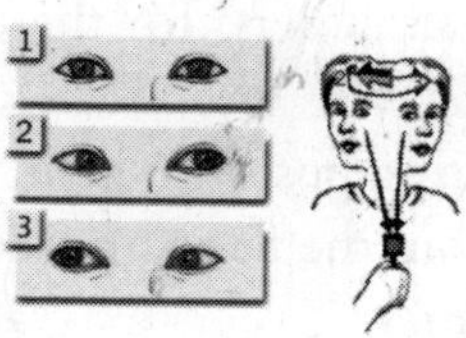

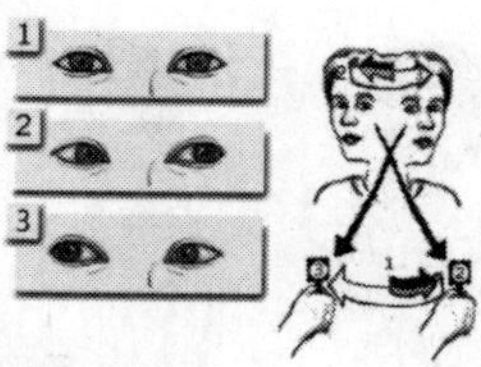

Head exercises

- With your eyes open, bend your head forwards, then backwards, 20 times. Start slowly at first, then speed up.

- With your eyes open, turn your head from side to side 20 times. Start slowly at first, then speed up.
- As the dizziness reduces, repeat the head exercises with your eyes closed.

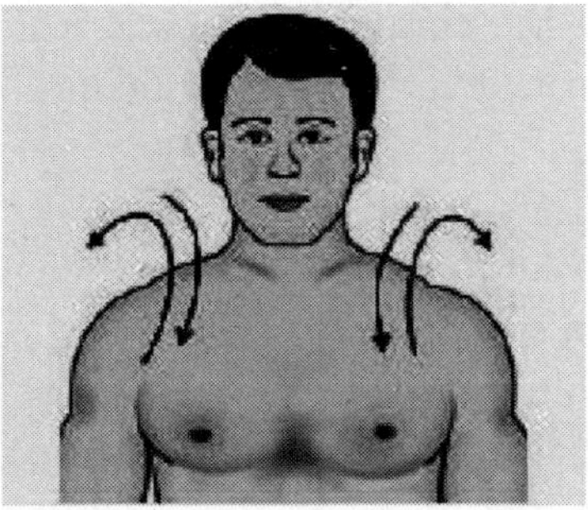

Sitting exercises

- Shrug your shoulders 20 times.
- Turn your shoulders to the right and left 20 times.
- From the sitting position, bend down and pick up objects from the floor, and sit back up again. Repeat 20 times.

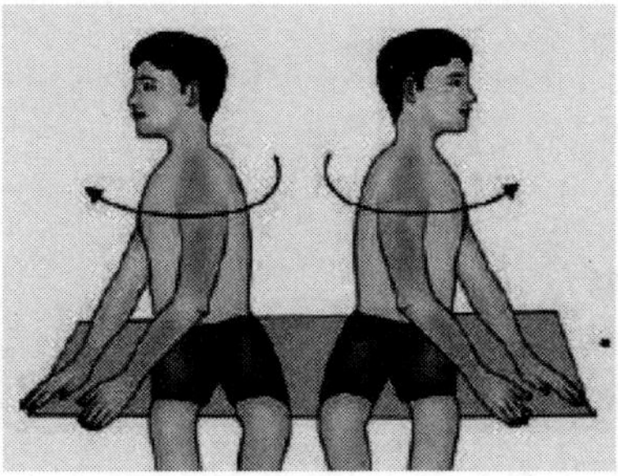

Standing exercises

- Move from sitting to standing up, and back again, with your eyes open, 20 times.
- Repeat with eyes closed.
- Throw a small ball from one hand to the other, above eye level, 20 times.
- Throw the ball from hand to hand at knee level, 20 times.
- Turn around 360 degrees on the spot, eyes open.
- Repeat with eyes closed.
- As vertigo lessens, speed up.

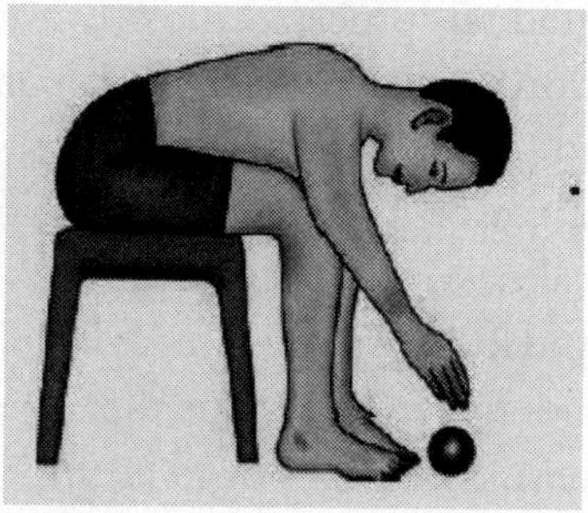

Moving about exercises (special caution advised)

- Walk across the floor with your eyes open 20 times.
- Repeat with eyes closed.
- Walk up and down a slope with your eyes open 20 times.
- Repeat with eyes closed.
- Walk up and down steps 20 times with your eyes open.
- Repeat with eyes closed.

- Any game or exercise that involves stooping, turning, bending, stretching and hand-eye coordination—for example bowling, tennis—is good for improving your balance.

Q3: My uncle is suffering from chronic kidney disease and also had a bypass surgery for heart four years ago. Nowadays, his muscles are grossly wasted. Despite being under constant medical care he looks very weak. Why?

The loss of muscle mass is called Sarcopenia and is normally a gradual process, mostly attributed to lack of nutrition and advancing age, comorbidities like heart and kidney ailment. Lack of exercises also become a reason for reduced muscle mass and generalised weakness.

Being a heart and kidney patient for long, obviously he would have undergone enormous dietary restrictions of fat and protein. And now not so healthy and active, it is but natural to have a compromised musculature. Also your uncle must be indoors most of the time, leading to deficiency of vitamin D, another big cause of poor muscles.

So, to have good muscle mass, regular exercises, adequate nutrition with protein intake 1-2 gm/kg body weight per day in addition to cereals, fruits and vegetables are must. There is a wrong perception that only non-vegetarian food can improve the muscle mass.

As medication, vitamin D and anabolic steroids are given. Some new medicines are under research but yet to pass clinical trials. In old age, anyway, one loses 1-2% muscle mass per year after 50 and may be up to 3% per year after 70.

Q4: My mother was complaining of muscle pain mainly in calf and of tiredness. The doctor said it is chronic fatigue syndrome. What is it?

Your mother may be a case of 'chronic fatigue syndrome' which can manifest as group of symptoms like muscle pain, tiredness, headaches, joint pains without swelling, loss of sleep and memory etc. If these symptoms persist for more than few months, then it can be labeled as chronic fatigue syndrome. Usually, muscle carnitine deficiency is the root cause and usually diagnosis is by exclusion of other causes rather than a positive one. Medication (levocarnitine) and psychotherapy are usually given by doctors and it works well.

Q5: I have seen certain small height (dwarfs) in circus and outside, do they have normal life?

The condition is rare, say 1 in 25,000 where growth is stunted; it is a genetic variation and has nothing to do with mothers' diet etc. The intelligence in achondoplasia people is normal but child bearing is usually not possible in females.

Q6: My wife has had no injury but keeps on having pain right on the front bone of chest. It does not settle with pain killers. What to do?

The front bone of chest is called sternum and ribs from this go back to spine. The junction of rib to sternum can have swelling/inflammation pain and the disease is called Tietz disease. The localised area of pain usually doesn't improve with medicines and local steroid injection is a very helpful treatment.

Rarely, at these joints tuberculosis can also happen, which is ascertained by strong suspicion, blood tests, MRI and if confirmed, anti-TB drugs will cure it after a prolonged therapy of 12 to 18 months.

Sometimes it is part of general body aches and pains, having more to do with psychology and less with pathology.

Q7: Is infection in a bone curable? My classmate is a perennial absentee on account of infection in leg which recurs again and again despite surgeries.

Yes, infection in bone can be rooted out and your classmate can live a normal life. Infection in bone is either through blood origin, when it travels from throat, urinary tract, stomach etc or it can be of local origin post injury or operation in bone and is called Osteomylitis. Usually the blood-born infection is more among children and less among adults while the post injury, post operation infection is more among adults and less among children.

Q9: I am a voluntary social worker at a government hospital and some educated patients ask us what is STEM cell therapy and how it can cure Arthritis and Spine problems?

Stem cell research definitely has lot of potential but not all medico legal aspects about it are clear. Stem cells are primitive cells already present in the body which can be made to differentiate or renew themselves over time and this science has been used for therapy of musculoskeletal disorders.

Q10: What is the simple height-weight criteria to remain healthy?

Body Mass index (BMI) is simple and standard.

Body Mass Index (BMI) = (W (Kg) / H (M2)

BMI	Classification
< 18.5	underweight
18.5–24.9	normal weight
25.0–29.9	overweight
30.0–34.9	class I obesity
35.0–39.9	class II obesity
≥ 40.0	class III obesity

Physiotherapy

Q1: I am a 57-year-old senior executive of a company and during my elaborate medical checkup, the clinicians discovered that my bones are osteoporotic. Can physiotherapy help in any way?

Well, if you are not having any complaints as such then physiotherapy gadgets are not required. The weight bearing exercises like walking, jogging, treadmill, weight training in gym are good enough for strengthening the bone stock.

Q2: We are a joint family having grandparents, parents and young members. Wherever any of us visits a physiotherapy centre for any musculoskeletal problem, they use different gadgets, many a times with no clear pattern. Is it that haphazard or there is a system?

All gadgets have a clearly defined role, it may so happen that the physiotherapist may apply a cocktail of machines to alleviate pain and improve function.

Few examples:

a) Ultrasonic Therapy (based on sound waves) is mostly used for neck and shoulder pain.

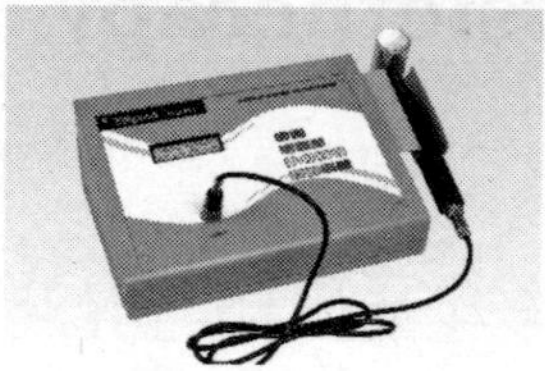

b) Short wave Diathermy (SWD) is deep heat. It is used for back and knees.

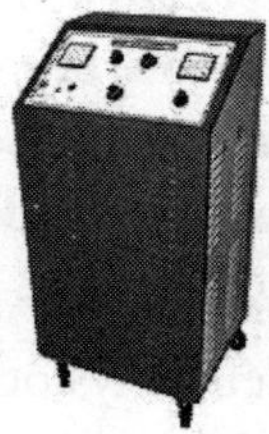

c) Muscle stimulator is used for strengthening weak muscles.

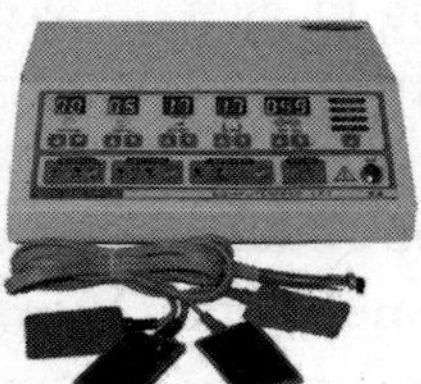

d) Nerve stimulator is used for improving current conduction in nerve.

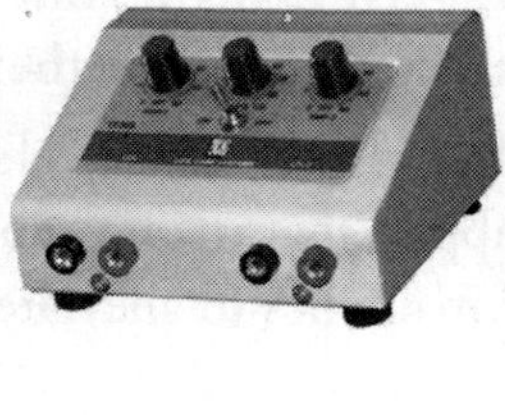

e) Intermittent pelvic traction machine is used for treating disc prolapse of back.

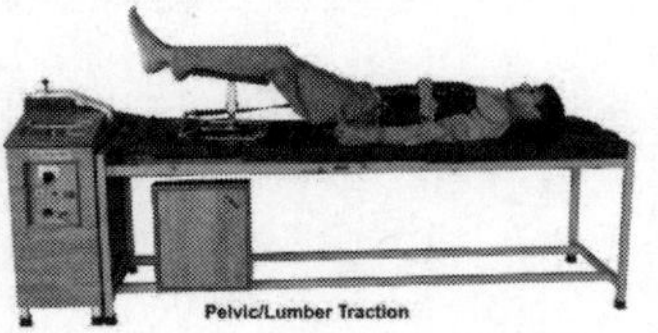

f) Continuous Passive Motion (CPM) is used to help knee bending with least pain.

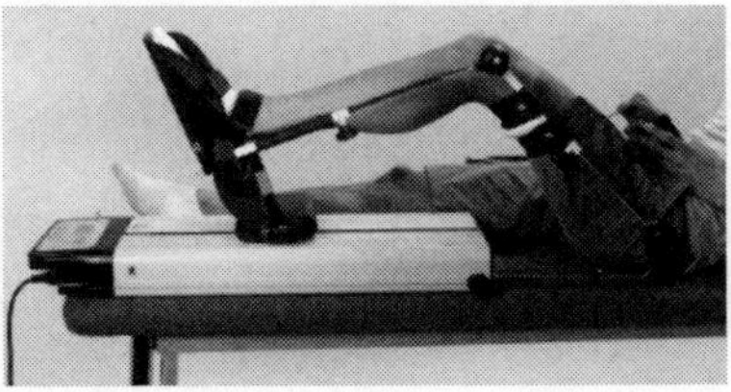

And there are many others. Usually, in one patient, two to three machines with additional exercises are used for better results.

Yoga

Q1: I am an executive of 46 years and these days I hear lot about yoga exercises in the media, are they really good for my muscles and bones?

Yoga is a type of weight bearing exercise where stress forces due to the weight of body plays against gravitational forces, resulting in strengthening the bones. Certainly, the stretching of muscles improves the tone, power and the body balance.

Other intense weight bearing exercises like sports and running do the same but they also damage cartilage and stress the joints and therefore require certain amount of discretion. Yoga is usually practiced with plant and milk based diets and high acid foods like meats, egg, fish and beverages are avoided.

Q2: With yoga exercises, are there any Dos and Don'ts, especially for particular disease profiles like backache, arthritic knees, cervical spondylitis etc?

Here are certain common 'Asanas' which have to be avoided in certain conditions:

a) Vakrasana (Tree pose) – avoided in knee pain

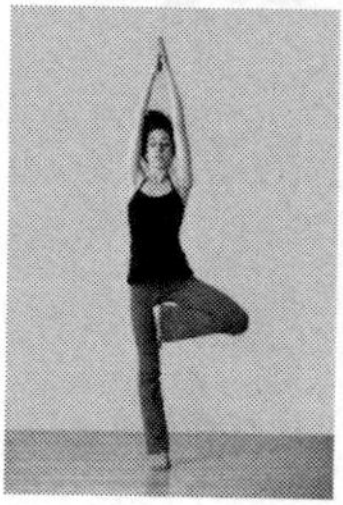

b) Utkatasana (Chair pose) – avoided in knee /back pain

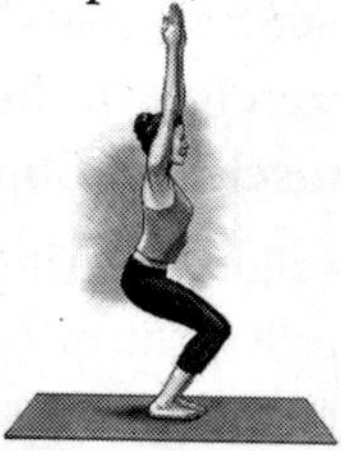

c) Bhujangasana (Cobra pose) – Safe

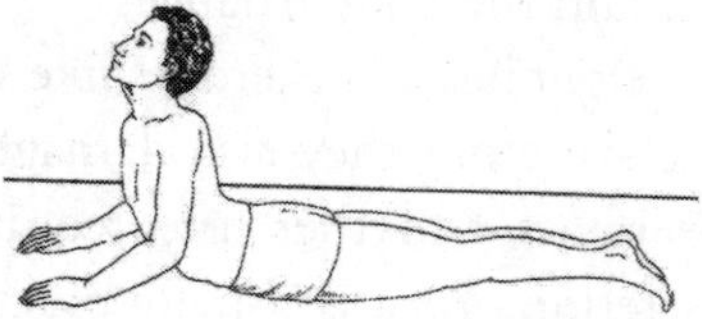

d) Setu bandha soonang asana (bridge pose) avoided in neck pain

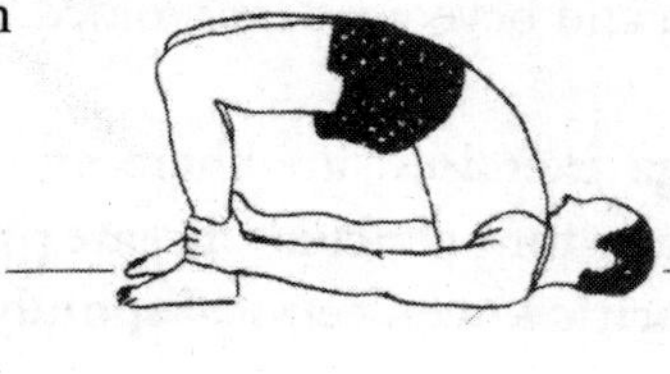

e) Virbhadrasana I (Warrior pose I) safe

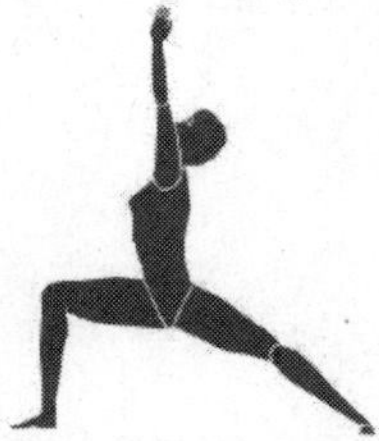

f) Virbhadrasana II (Warrior pose II) safe

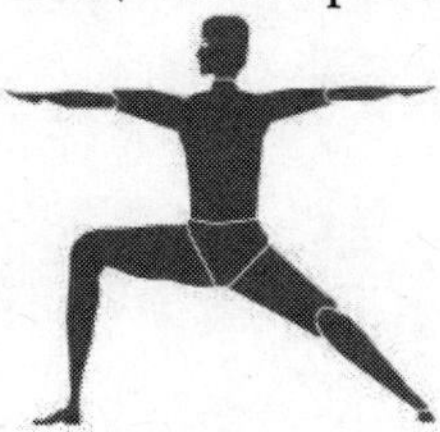

g) Sheershasana – avoid in neck pain

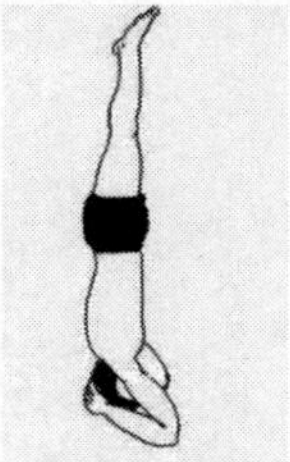

h) Padmasana – sitting with cross legs – avoid in knee pain

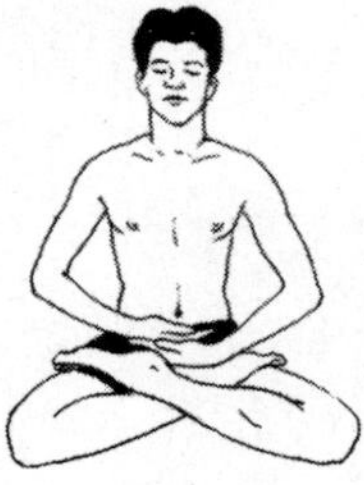

Cancer & Bone Tumours

Q1: Somebody may call it my ignorance but it came as a shocking news to me that bones can also have cancer. How far is it true in light of the fact that my maid's son is suspected of one at shoulder blade (back)?

Yes, bones are also prone to cancer and tumours which can be benign (non-cancerous) or malignant (cancerous). There are bone forming, cartilage forming or marrow tumours. In benign tumours growth is slow, limited, less dangerous but in malignant tumours growth is fast, aggressive and the spread is local as well as to other organs. Cancer tumour cells can easily spread to brain, lungs, spine etc mainly through blood.

In your maid's son's case chondrosarcoma tumour (from shoulder blade bone cartilage) should be ruled out by MRI and biopsy.

Q2: My office colleague's son, 15 years old male, had a large painful swelling at lower thigh. Now ortho surgeon suspects a tumour called osteosarcoma. Does the poor child have any future?

Yes, in this age group malignant tumour like osteosarcoma near the knee joint can be very dangerous. Earliest MRI, biopsy will confirm the diagnosis. Then Enblock excision surgery followed by endo prosthesis to make limb viable is provided. Chemotherapy (cancer medicines) usually follows. No doubt such a surgery is very traumatic. But it is very important to salvage the limb and life.

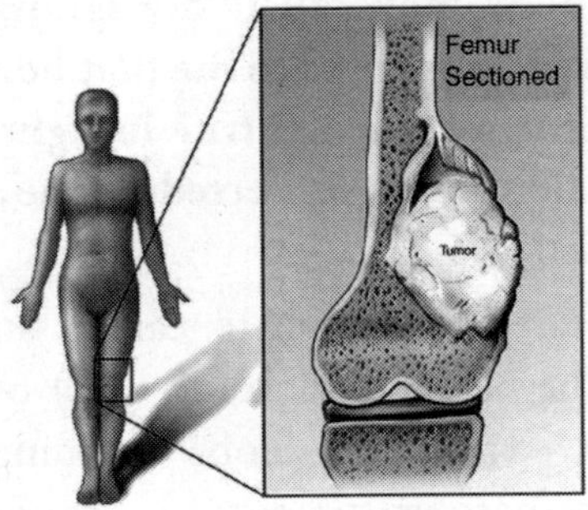

Q3: At what stage do we say that this child has poor prognosis?

Usually tumours are graded by orthopedics

1: a b

2: a b

3: a b

3 a/b are designated as having poor prognosis.

The patients of malignant tumours have approximately 5 to 10 years' life expectancy. Now, with better surgery, chemotherapy and radiotherapy life expectancy has improved. Especially for cases which are diagnosed at early stage.

Q4: My grandmother is a known case of cancer. Breast is under treatment but for last 6 weeks there is severe pain in hip area. The MRI shows cancer cells have spread in that area also. What is the remedy to this complex issue?

The spread of breast carcinoma to bones, especially pelvis is know. Usually radiotherapy sittings reduce pain very well. As far as cancer treatment is concerned, chemotherapy with advice of cancer specialist will be helpful. Similarly, secondary spread to bones can occur from primary cancer of kidney, prostrate etc.

Q5: Life gave a rude shock to our family when my aunt, 57, went to ortho-surgeon for treatment of severe low backache and was diagnosed with cancer after positive blood tests. Unbelievable because nothing was visible!

Your aunt's low backache and pelvis area pain, which may not be settling down with routine treatments must have been subjected to x-ray and blood tests. A cancer of bone marrow called multiple myeloma can be diagnosed from serum electrophoresis (blood) test showing myeloma proteins.

Now, she needs complete course of chemotherapy under strict surveillance. May be some radiotherapy too. If cancer has spread, prognosis is bad. Early diagnosis and early treatment is of great help.

Q6: Our watchman's wife who came from Nepal had a fracture below shoulder. Doctor said fracture is secondary to a cystic lesion which had weakened bone at the site, sounds surprising? Will it be cured?

Bone cyst, of various types may develop at the end of long bones. They are not cancerous but like a balloon, expand and weaken the walls of bone, ultimately leading to fracture.

If diagnosed at early stage of pain, bone cyst can be treated and fracture can be avoided because such pathological fractures (in unhealthy bone) are difficult to unite. Just curettage (scrapping the cavity) and fitting it with bone graft or bone cement cures the condition usually.

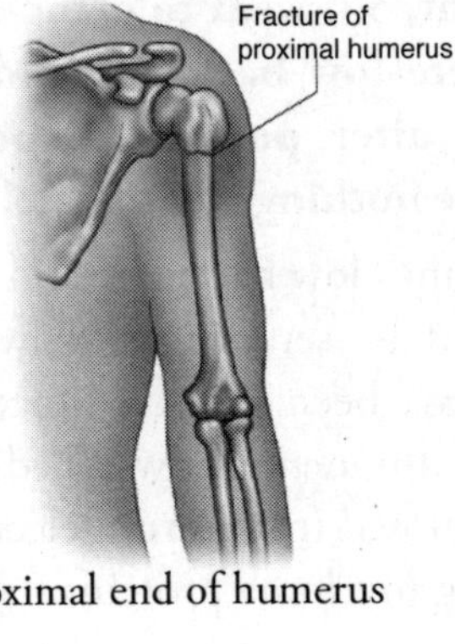

Cyst at the proximal end of humerus

Osteoporosis

Q1: How much alcohol is permissible, which is not detrimental to bone health?

Usually 30ml 3 times a week is safe limit as per some nutrition advisories.

Q2: My mother is regularly taking calcium for bones. Still, in the last week when her bone density was done, she was osteoporotic. Why?

Osteoporosis is weakening of bones (porous bones). Bone matrix is not only made of calcium and vitamin D but also of protein matrix. Your mother was consuming calcium which alone is not sufficient. As it is, chances of osteoporosis in women above 45 (ie. post-menopausal women) is one in three.

If her Dexa scan bone mineral density (BMD) score is less than (T score) -2.5 at spine, hips, wrist, then she needs anti-osteoporotic treatment. The treatment options are Ca, Vitamin D, anti-bone resorptives and hormone treatment like pteriperatide. The antibone resorptive agents like bisphosphonates stop the destruction (catabolism) of bone and can be taken for 2 to 5 years, along with Ca and Vitamin D. While pteriperatide is more expensive therapy, it has anabolic properties, ie. bone forming action and this can be taken for 1½ years.

Q3: My father, 68 years, is an ex-army officer and was having backache. The doctor advised BMD test. Strange! Do men have osteoporosis?

Yes, men do have osteoporosis and the incidence is one in five after 50 years of age. Doctor has rightly advised bone density because weakness is the reason for fragility, collapse or fracture of vertebrae in spine, the major cause of pain. Many a times patient doesn't even have any precipitate history of fall or injury. So do not get surprised if X-Ray shows collapse of vertebrae and BMD proves osteoporosis, this calls for complete treatment.

Q4: Both my parents were diagnosed with osteoporosis. How do I save myself?

Osteoporosis is a silent disease and doesn't have any symptoms till there is some fracture of bone. The genetic factor is something you can't help but you can prevent weakness of bones to a great extent by exercises, diet, sun exposure, calcium, Vitamin D intake and cutting down on risk factors.

Q5: What diet should I take for strong bones?

Dairy foods such as whole or skimmed milk, curd and cheese are rich in calcium that is easily absorbed by the body. Some calcium-fortified beverages (such as orange juice or soya milk) may contain as much calcium as milk. Certain vegetables and fruits (eg. banana, beans) also provide calcium, as does fish containing bones.

Too much salt and caffeine may increase the loss of calcium through the urine. Calcium content of some common foods:

Food	Calcium (Mg)
Milk	297 mg/cup
Curd	300 mg/cup
Cheese	155 mg/cup
Soya bean	90 mg/cup
Green Vegetables	200 mg/cup

If you consume this kind of diet in a wise and judicious way, certainly it will be very helpful for strong bones.

Q6: Do you think I should be scared of osteoporosis, being a female of 40?

Scared? No. But definitely weak bones lead to fracture of hip, shoulder, wrist, vertebrae (back) ribs as a result of minor trauma. These are called fragility fractures and are very common. So, prevention and early diagnosis of osteoporosis is of great value.

Q7: I am a male of 35 years. Although I go for daily morning walk, please suggest me some exercises which are best to prevent osteoporosis?

There are two types of exercises that are important for building and maintaining bone density: weight-bearing and muscle-strengthening exercises.

Weight-bearing Exercises

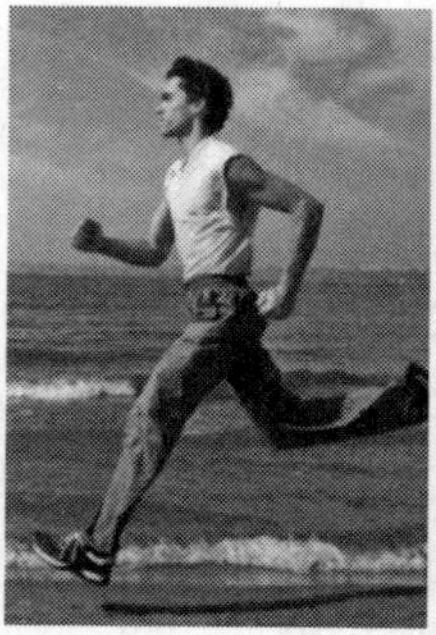

Running

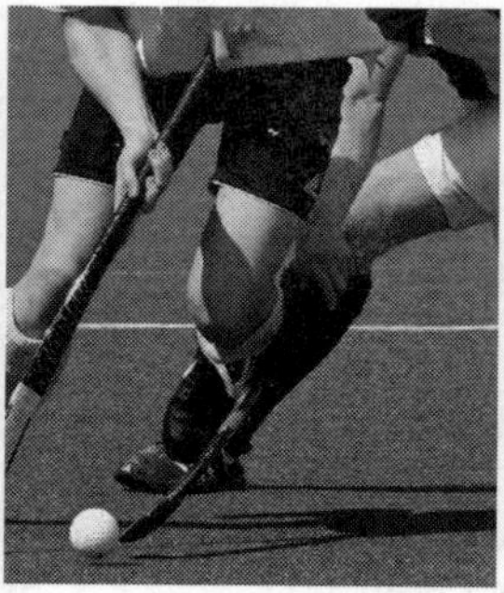

Hockey

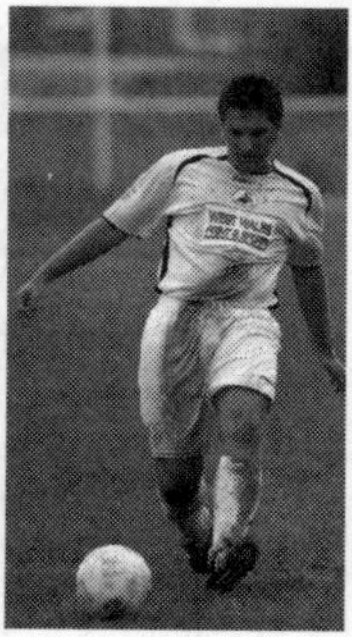

Football

These exercises include activities that make you move against gravity while staying upright. Weight-bearing exercises can be high-impact or low-impact.

Examples of high-impact weight-bearing exercises are dancing, doing high-impact aerobics, jogging/running, field games like Hockey, Football, Tennis etc. Low-impact weight-bearing exercises can also help keep bones strong and are a safe alternative if you cannot do high-impact exercises. **Examples of low-**

impact weight-bearing exercises are doing low-impact aerobics, using step machines, fast walking on a treadmill or outside in the park.

Muscle-strengthening Exercises

These exercises include activities where you move your body, a weight or some other resistance against gravity. They are also known as resistance exercises and include lifting weights, using elastic exercise bands, using weight machines, lifting your own body weight, functional movements such as standing and rising up on your toes. They are possible while playing and in the gym.

Q8: What are the risk factors in osteoporosis which I need to avoid?

Alcohol and smoking have detrimental effect. Diseases like diabetes, hypothyroid, epilepsy (convulsions), gastritis (on antacids), stomach food absorption problems such as Crohn's disease, irritable bowel syndrome and frequent diarrhea can impede with absorption of Ca and Vitamin D, leading to weak bones. Sedentary life itself is a risk factor.

Q9: Should I get my son, 10 years old, checked for osteoporosis?

No, it is generally found that osteoporosis manifests in adulthood and children don't suffer from it.

Q10: My brother's wife, post-delivery, has been suffering a lot of bone pains; in her last delivery it was less severe. Can't she work at all?

Your brother's wife is most likely suffering from Osteomalacia. It is a disease with gross deficiency of Calcium and Vitamin D. Post delivery, in the lactating mothers, calcium is mobilised from bones and the requirement of patient is very high and in such cases, Osteomalacia can happen. Indeed, it is a very painful condition, the aches are generally around pelvis, hips and spine. She must be having some problem after first delivery also, but the second pregnancy without fair interval of 3 to 4 years must have precipitated her pain in a big way.

Fortunately, she will immediately improve (in 2 to 3 months) if proper Calcium and Vitamin D therapy is done and proper diet is taken. Yes, breast feeding needs to be stopped in severe cases and the baby is switched over to top milk.

Q11: My mother is suffering from arthritis and osteoporosis both, what is the difference? Lot of confusion.

Indeed, there can be confusion especially if both ailments exist in the same patient. If we put it in simple words, the pain and swelling in joints like knee, elbows, and wrists in your mother's case is because of arthritis; while the weakness of bones like thigh long bone, arm bone, back vertebrae etc is due to osteoporosis. Both are completely different ailments but the confusion is only because, both are related to bones and joints. Even the treatments are completely different. It is like confusing bronchial asthma and TB of lungs because they are happening in the same organ. Best way to fight confusion is awareness and information about twin conditions.

Q12: My wife, 50 years old, has been osteoporotic, can we do something at home to help her?

Yes, you can ensure regular intake of milk 300ml or milk products, fruits like banana, apple, pineapple, veggies like broccoli. Incorporating tofu and yogurt in diet is a good idea. No doubt, if she can have fish like salmon, a very rich source of Calcium and Vitamin D, it will be of help. In addition to this, if she can go for a morning/evening walk of 1 hour daily, it will be fantastic.

Q13a: My grandson is only four and his legs are going apart visibly. Is it calcium deficiency?

This disease is called rickets and is responsible for deformities of legs called knock-knees or bow-legs. Reason is calcium and vitamin D deficiency.

The Ca and Vitamin-D deficiency can be corrected by replenishing with heavy doses at initial stage; also splints to keep limbs in correct position are used for day and night. Additionally, the child should be given Vitamin-D oil massage followed by 40 min of sun bath. In children above 8 years, where the efforts of cure have either not been done or have failed, surgery is the option. Here the deformed bones are cut in a way that they unite in corrected manner; usually recovery period is two to three months.

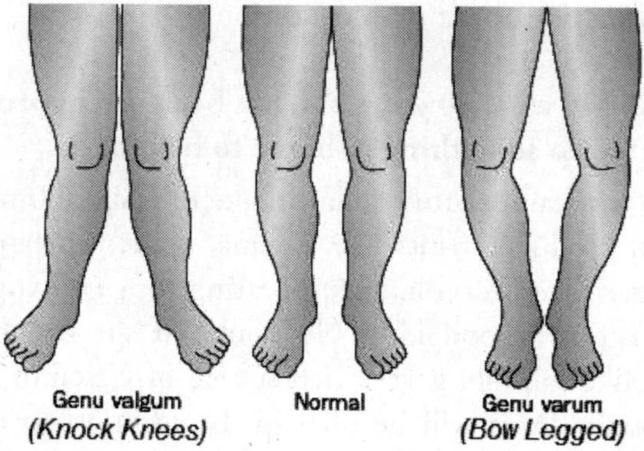

Q13b: Is it possible to correct the alignment of the legs without cutting bone?

Yes, it is possible by surgery called Epiphysiodesis. in this the growing end of lower thigh bone (femur) is stapled or plated in such away that the growth of thigh is allowed only on outer side and thus gradually over a period of 1 year automatically leg which is going out comes in the normal position.

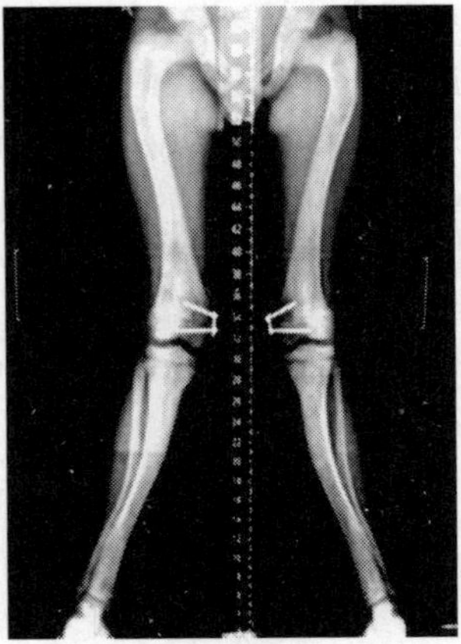

Q14: My wife is pregnant and taking calcium and iron tablets, should she take vitamin D also?

Vitamin D Consumption is not advisable in pregnant women without proven deficiency. Also, the same holds true in nursing mothers because vitamin D passes into breast milk.

Q15: My mother was regularly taking calcium and vitamin D and for a different problem she visited a doctor and he prescribed heavy doses of vitamin D. Now she is having headache, fatigue, weakness, nausea and vomiting. Reason?

Well, these symptoms are adverse actions of vitamin D and are reversible once vitamin D is withdrawn but consult a Endocrinologist to find out about renal damage.

Q16: Can there be hyper vitaminosis of Vitamin D ?

Yes, It is possible, especially in kidney-compromised patients. Hyper vitaminosis may lead to heart problems also. Therefore, one has to be watchful about over dosage. If the blood level is normal, only maintenance dose of 60k units once a month is more than enough. Visit a specialist and clarify in case of doubt.

Miscellaneous

Q1: I am a woman of 45, having giddiness and vertigo for the last few months. My family physician gave some medicines but they are not helping much. What to do?

Giddiness/vertigo is a very common problem and has many underlying causes, but a large section of patients fall into the category of Benign Postural Vertigo (BPV) where there is no clear-cut positive disease finding. You can have vertigo for a short period, say 5-10 min and which may disappear without any medication but to reappear again. This shakes the confidence of the patient. Answer is symptomatic anti-vertigo treatment and regular exercises dedicated to vertigo, also known as 'Vertigo Rehab Regime'. Gradually, problems will settle down.

The other kind of vertigo patients may be due to cervical spondylitis (neck degeneration changes).They improve with cervical collar, temporary halting of exercises and/or anti-vertigo medicines. Once vertigo is controlled, they can renew neck exercises.

Some of the patients who have ear problem, cochlear disturbances, need to be checked by ENT surgeon for middle ear problems and usually settle down with a mixture of above mentioned treatments on a prolonged basis.

Last but not the least, refractory error (vision defects) should be ruled out. Also hypertension needs to be taken care of. It is advisable that patients of vertigo should avoid adventure rides, jerky circular dancing and similar activities.

Q2: What is vertigo rehabilitation regime?

Vertigo is a particular form of dizziness or giddiness. Rather than just feeling faint or light headed, it is an illusion of motion. The sufferer feels as though they, or their surroundings, are turning, spinning, falling, or some other form of movement when in fact they are not. Like sea-sickness, vertigo is often accompanied by nausea and vomiting.

Once you have identified dizziness-provoking movements, you can begin an exercise programme to repeat those movements to help you to achieve vestibular compensation. It's important to repeat them at least five times in a row and twice a day. If you find there are several different movements that make you dizzy, pick two to work on at a time. Once you no longer experience dizziness in response to these movements, add two more. Don't try to do exercises for more than two movements at a time.

Following are the common exercises which can be done. You can take a therapist's guidance initially if you wish:

Eye exercises

- Look up and down 20 times. Start slowly at first, then speed up.
- Look from one side to the other 20 times. Start slowly at first, then speed up.
- Hold up one finger at arm's length. Focus on it. Move it slowly in towards you and out again 20 times.

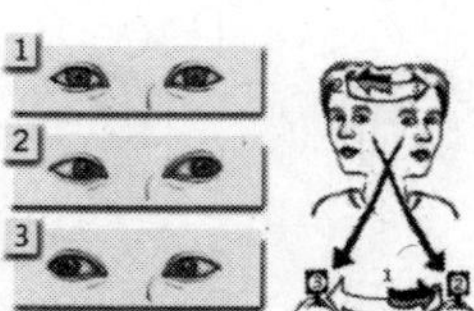

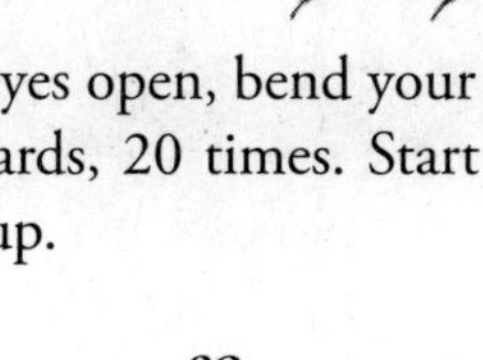

Head exercises

- With your eyes open, bend your head forwards, then backwards, 20 times. Start slowly at first, then speed up.

- With your eyes open, turn your head from side to side 20 times. Start slowly at first, then speed up.
- As the dizziness reduces, repeat the head exercises with your eyes closed.

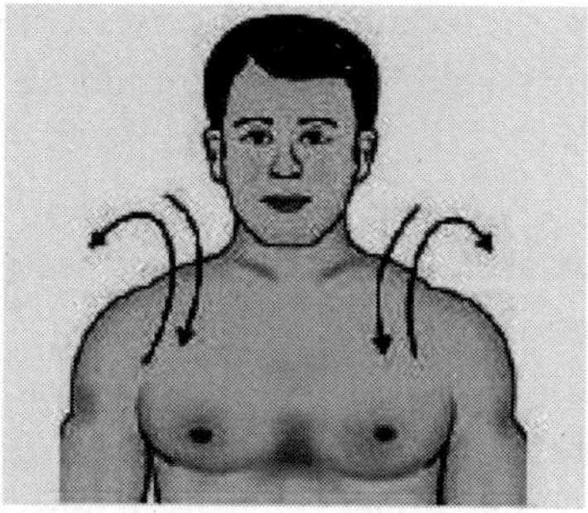

Sitting exercises

- Shrug your shoulders 20 times.
- Turn your shoulders to the right and left 20 times.
- From the sitting position, bend down and pick up objects from the floor, and sit back up again. Repeat 20 times.

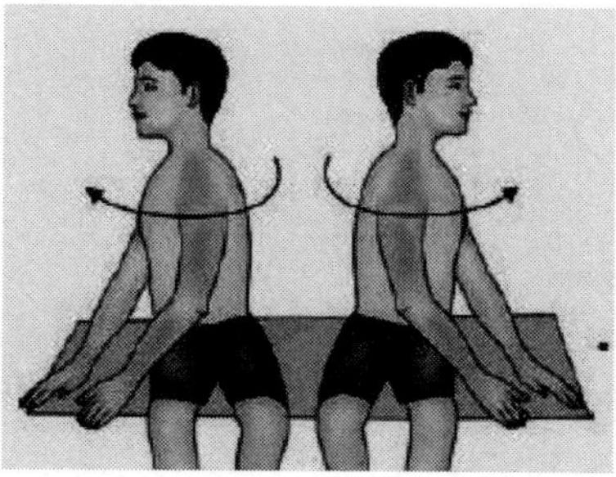

Standing exercises

- Move from sitting to standing up, and back again, with your eyes open, 20 times.
- Repeat with eyes closed.
- Throw a small ball from one hand to the other, above eye level, 20 times.
- Throw the ball from hand to hand at knee level, 20 times.
- Turn around 360 degrees on the spot, eyes open.
- Repeat with eyes closed.
- As vertigo lessens, speed up.

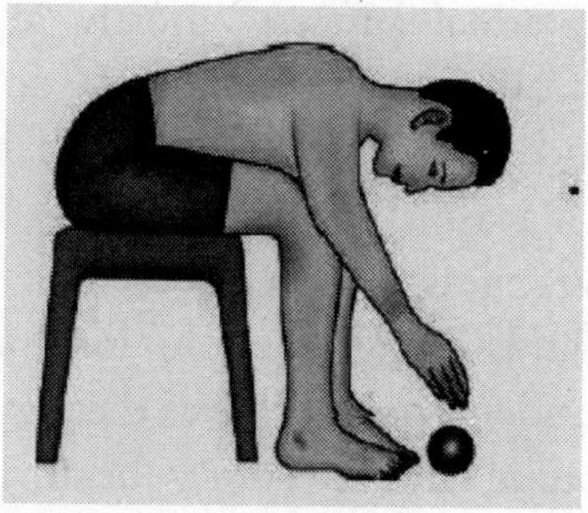

Moving about exercises (special caution advised)

- Walk across the floor with your eyes open 20 times.
- Repeat with eyes closed.
- Walk up and down a slope with your eyes open 20 times.
- Repeat with eyes closed.
- Walk up and down steps 20 times with your eyes open.
- Repeat with eyes closed.

- Any game or exercise that involves stooping, turning, bending, stretching and hand-eye coordination—for example bowling, tennis—is good for improving your balance.

Q3: My uncle is suffering from chronic kidney disease and also had a bypass surgery for heart four years ago. Nowadays, his muscles are grossly wasted. Despite being under constant medical care he looks very weak. Why?

The loss of muscle mass is called Sarcopenia and is normally a gradual process, mostly attributed to lack of nutrition and advancing age, comorbidities like heart and kidney ailment. Lack of exercises also become a reason for reduced muscle mass and generalised weakness.

Being a heart and kidney patient for long, obviously he would have undergone enormous dietary restrictions of fat and protein. And now not so healthy and active, it is but natural to have a compromised musculature. Also your uncle must be indoors most of the time, leading to deficiency of vitamin D, another big cause of poor muscles.

So, to have good muscle mass, regular exercises, adequate nutrition with protein intake 1-2 gm/kg body weight per day in addition to cereals, fruits and vegetables are must. There is a wrong perception that only non-vegetarian food can improve the muscle mass.

As medication, vitamin D and anabolic steroids are given. Some new medicines are under research but yet to pass clinical trials. In old age, anyway, one loses 1-2% muscle mass per year after 50 and may be up to 3% per year after 70.

Q4: My mother was complaining of muscle pain mainly in calf and of tiredness. The doctor said it is chronic fatigue syndrome. What is it?

Your mother may be a case of 'chronic fatigue syndrome' which can manifest as group of symptoms like muscle pain, tiredness, headaches, joint pains without swelling, loss of sleep and memory etc. If these symptoms persist for more than few months, then it can be labeled as chronic fatigue syndrome. Usually, muscle carnitine deficiency is the root cause and usually diagnosis is by exclusion of other causes rather than a positive one. Medication (levocarnitine) and psychotherapy are usually given by doctors and it works well.

Q5: I have seen certain small height (dwarfs) in circus and outside, do they have normal life?

The condition is rare, say 1 in 25,000 where growth is stunted; it is a genetic variation and has nothing to do with mothers' diet etc. The intelligence in achondoplasia people is normal but child bearing is usually not possible in females.

Q6: My wife has had no injury but keeps on having pain right on the front bone of chest. It does not settle with pain killers. What to do?

The front bone of chest is called sternum and ribs from this go back to spine. The junction of rib to sternum can have swelling/inflammation pain and the disease is called Tietz disease. The localised area of pain usually doesn't improve with medicines and local steroid injection is a very helpful treatment.

Rarely, at these joints tuberculosis can also happen, which is ascertained by strong suspicion, blood tests, MRI and if confirmed, anti-TB drugs will cure it after a prolonged therapy of 12 to 18 months.

Sometimes it is part of general body aches and pains, having more to do with psychology and less with pathology.

Q7: Is infection in a bone curable? My classmate is a perennial absentee on account of infection in leg which recurs again and again despite surgeries.

Yes, infection in bone can be rooted out and your classmate can live a normal life. Infection in bone is either through blood origin, when it travels from throat, urinary tract, stomach etc or it can be of local origin post injury or operation in bone and is called Osteomylitis. Usually the blood-born infection is more among children and less among adults while the post injury, post operation infection is more among adults and less among children.

In your classmate's case osteomyelitis needs surgery in the form of dead bone removal (sequestrectomy), saucerisation (saucer shape given to the infected bone part) and also these days, an antibiotic loaded, biodegradable small bone cement ball/s can be put at the site. All this will most likely eradicate infection from there in six weeks' time. Remember, it is a difficult situation and there are no guaranteed results.

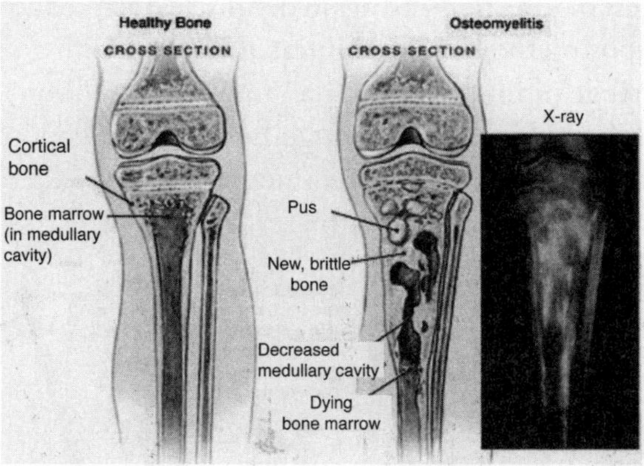

Q8: My father is 57 and had a titanium rod fixation after a fracture in right thigh bone, 6 weeks later pus started pouring and the fracture is not united. The family is stressed out, what is the cause?

It is unfortunate that your father's thigh bone nail got infected despite a proper surgery. Nevertheless, the situation has to be tackled. Usually with infection, union of fracture gets delayed and it is difficult to eradicate infection completely. The best option is, letting the fracture unite and suppress the infection with antibiotics; if fracture unites even in 6 months' time, then implant (nail) is removed. But if the infection doesn't allow union, then there is no solution and two stage surgery needs to be performed.

Stage 1-Removal of nail, cleaning the fracture area of infection and putting external fixation.

Stage 2-Removal of external fixation after complete arrest of infection and again definitive open reduction (exposing the bone)and internal fixation with a plate (change of implant from nail to plate better now).

All these things sound tough but they are important for your father's healthy movement and after an ordeal, life is back to normal.

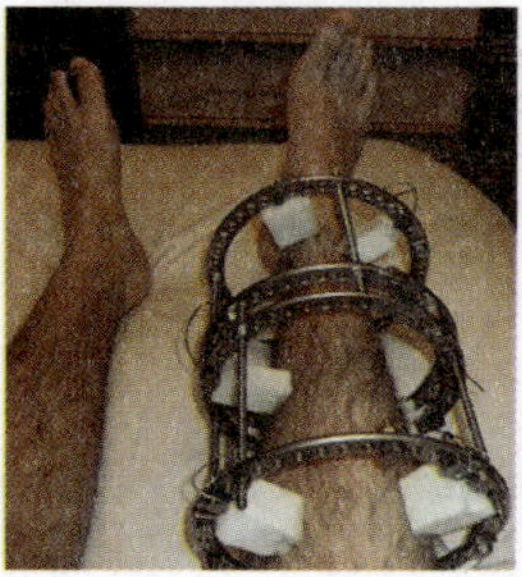

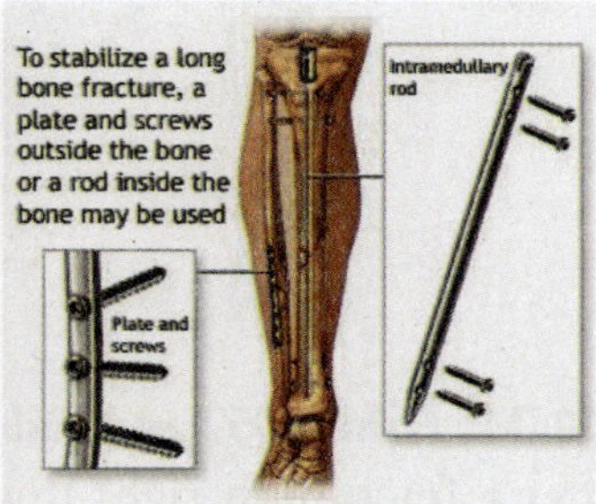

Photo of fixation

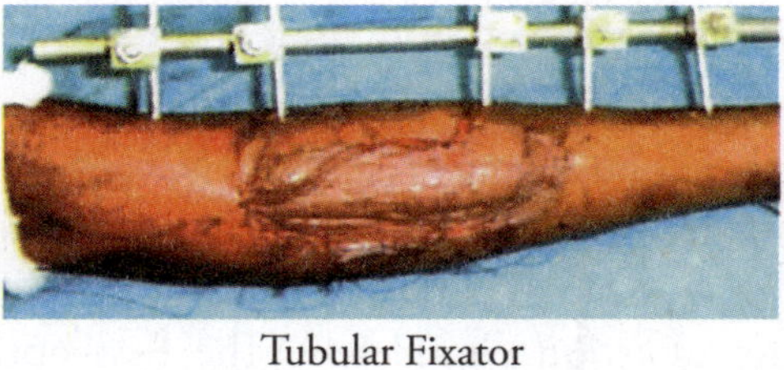

Tubular Fixator

Q9: I am a voluntary social worker at a government hospital and some educated patients ask us what is STEM cell therapy and how it can cure Arthritis and Spine problems?

Stem cell research definitely has lot of potential but not all medico legal aspects about it are clear. Stem cells are primitive cells already present in the body which can be made to differentiate or renew themselves over time and this science has been used for therapy of musculoskeletal disorders.

Q10: What is the simple height-weight criteria to remain healthy?

Body Mass index (BMI) is simple and standard.
Body Mass Index (BMI) = (W (Kg) / H (M2)

BMI	Classification
< 18.5	underweight
18.5–24.9	normal weight
25.0–29.9	overweight
30.0–34.9	class I obesity
35.0–39.9	class II obesity
≥ 40.0	class III obesity

Physiotherapy

Q1: I am a 57-year-old senior executive of a company and during my elaborate medical checkup, the clinicians discovered that my bones are osteoporotic. Can physiotherapy help in any way?

Well, if you are not having any complaints as such then physiotherapy gadgets are not required. The weight bearing exercises like walking, jogging, treadmill, weight training in gym are good enough for strengthening the bone stock.

Q2: We are a joint family having grandparents, parents and young members. Wherever any of us visits a physiotherapy centre for any musculoskeletal problem, they use different gadgets, many a times with no clear pattern. Is it that haphazard or there is a system?

All gadgets have a clearly defined role, it may so happen that the physiotherapist may apply a cocktail of machines to alleviate pain and improve function.

Few examples:

a) Ultrasonic Therapy (based on sound waves) is mostly used for neck and shoulder pain.

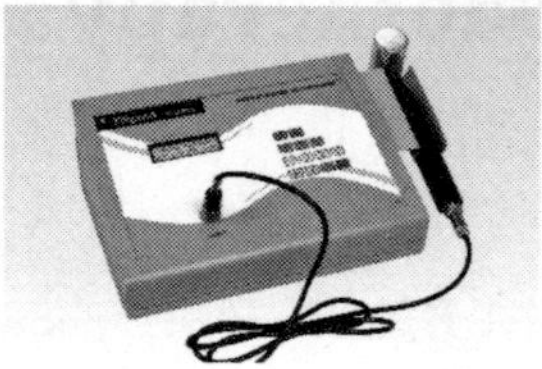

b) Short wave Diathermy (SWD) is deep heat. It is used for back and knees.

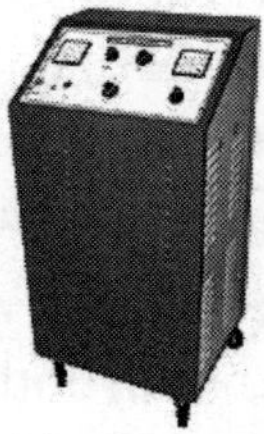

c) Muscle stimulator is used for strengthening weak muscles.

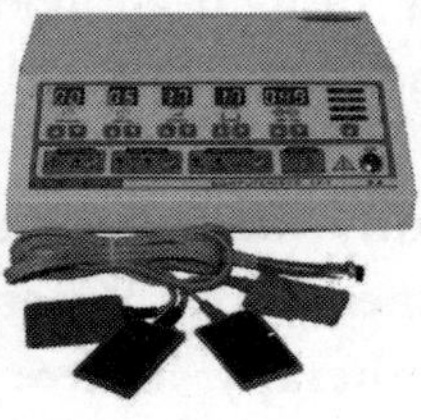

d) Nerve stimulator is used for improving current conduction in nerve.

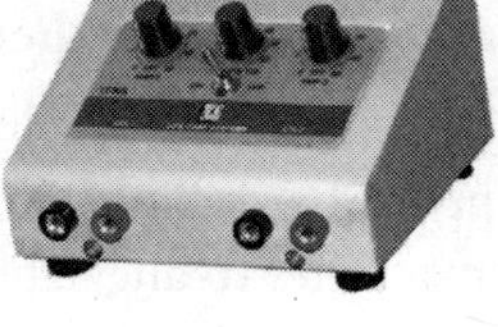

e) Intermittent pelvic traction machine is used for treating disc prolapse of back.

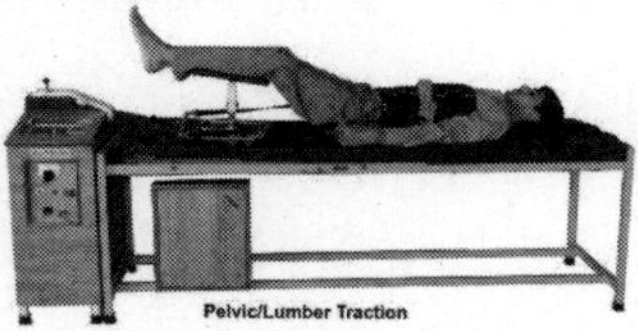

Pelvic/Lumber Traction

f) Continuous Passive Motion (CPM) is used to help knee bending with least pain.

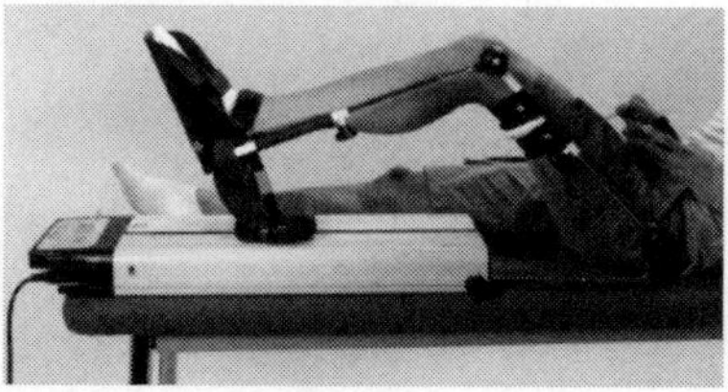

And there are many others. Usually, in one patient, two to three machines with additional exercises are used for better results.

Yoga

Q1: I am an executive of 46 years and these days I hear lot about yoga exercises in the media, are they really good for my muscles and bones?

Yoga is a type of weight bearing exercise where stress forces due to the weight of body plays against gravitational forces, resulting in strengthening the bones. Certainly, the stretching of muscles improves the tone, power and the body balance.

Other intense weight bearing exercises like sports and running do the same but they also damage cartilage and stress the joints and therefore require certain amount of discretion. Yoga is usually practiced with plant and milk based diets and high acid foods like meats, egg, fish and beverages are avoided.

Q2: With yoga exercises, are there any Dos and Don'ts, especially for particular disease profiles like backache, arthritic knees, cervical spondylitis etc?

Here are certain common 'Asanas' which have to be avoided in certain conditions:

a) Vakrasana (Tree pose) – avoided in knee pain

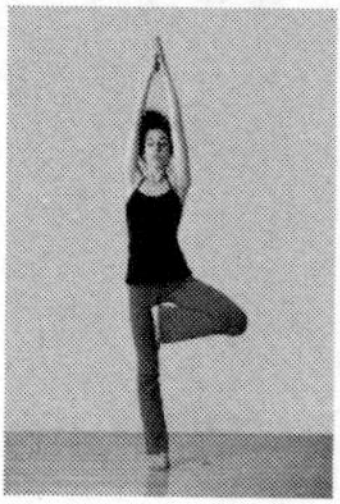

b) Utkatasana (Chair pose) – avoided in knee /back pain

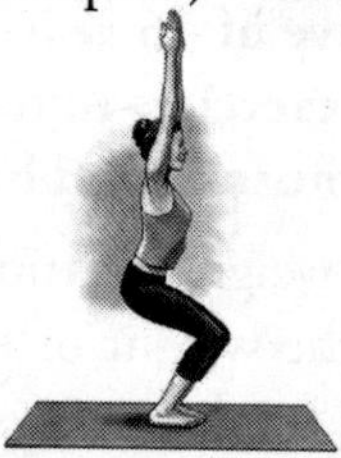

c) Bhujangasana (Cobra pose) – Safe

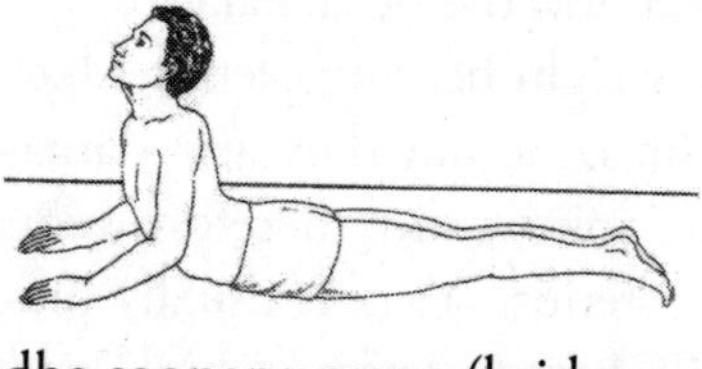

d) Setu bandha soonang asana (bridge pose) avoided in neck pain

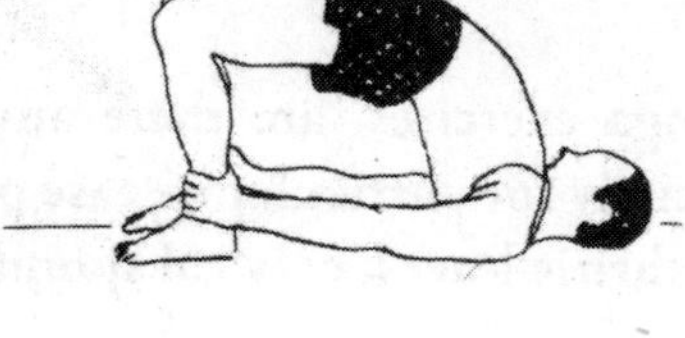

e) Virbhadrasana I (Warrior pose I) safe

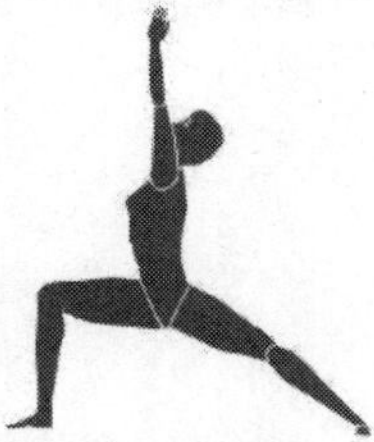

f) Virbhadrasana II (Warrior pose II) safe

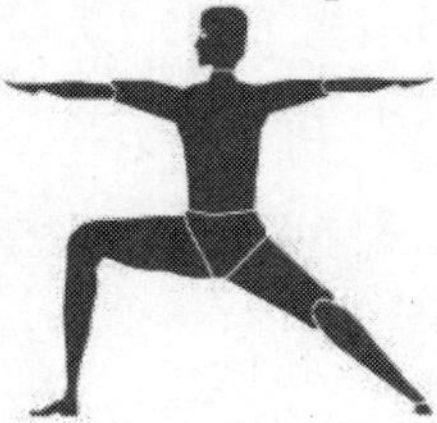

g) Sheershasana – avoid in neck pain

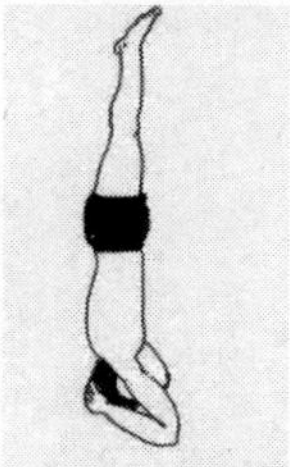

h) Padmasana – sitting with cross legs – avoid in knee pain

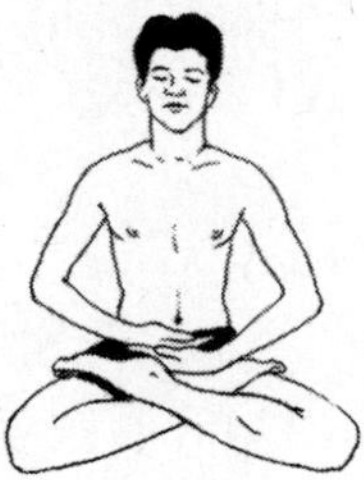

Gymming

Q1: I started weight training in gym and my coach said to put on a back support belt and wrist band, why?

The back support belt (lumber corset) is a must for weight training in gym otherwise there is a fair chance of you having disc prolapse and sciatica. This will require long rest and physiotherapy and you will have to stop weight training.

As far as wrist support band is concerned, don't think it is just a cosmetic appendage of smartness put on by tennis or golf players, rather it is a compressive device to hold your tendons and ligaments at the time of stress during weight lifting also. This will prevent snapping of these vital tissues.

Q2: Please advise as to how to avoid injuries in gym, which I am prone to.

- Technique should be right. Respect the integrity of muscle by not twisting or turning the muscles unnaturally, especially during weight training.
- Don't try too much weight which your muscles are not able to support and control.
- A point of total failure or giving way during bench press, can harm the gymnast.
- Warm up before actual exercises, is a must.
- Don't be hypoglycemic (reduced sugar to brain) and asphyxiated (struggling for breathing).
- Don't exercise too heavily while fasting.
- Light and regular workout are good for cutting on obesity.
- Don't talk to other gymnast friends or workout with divided attention. It may be cause of injury.
- Physical training is more like meditation.
- Don't forget, you know your limits better than others.
- Musical songs or visuals on TV may distract you, especially on treadmill, leading to fall. Sober instrumental music is preferable.

Q3: What are the dos and don'ts in relation to gymming gadgets?

SQUAT STATION

Dos: Good for strengthening of thigh and pelvic muscles around hips.

Don'ts: Not advisable for people with hip and knee early arthritis (caution for gymmers above 45).

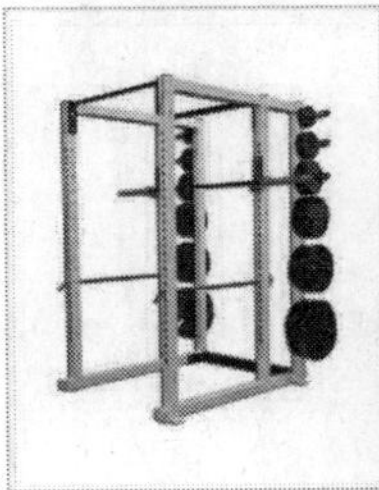

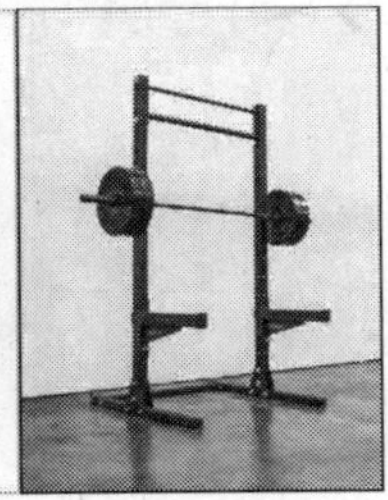

BENCH PRESS

Dos: Great exercise for forearm (extensor and flexor group). Arm and shoulder (biceps and triceps) girdle muscles (deltoid, pectorals).

Don'ts: Never do without prior muscle buildup with dumbbells and other shoulder girdle exercise.

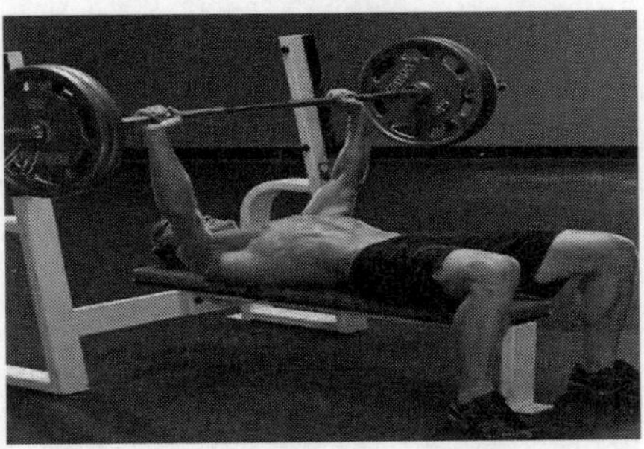

INCLINE BENCH PRESS

Dos: Similar but tougher version of bench press.

Don'ts: To avoid sudden weight drop, helper at head end is advisable.

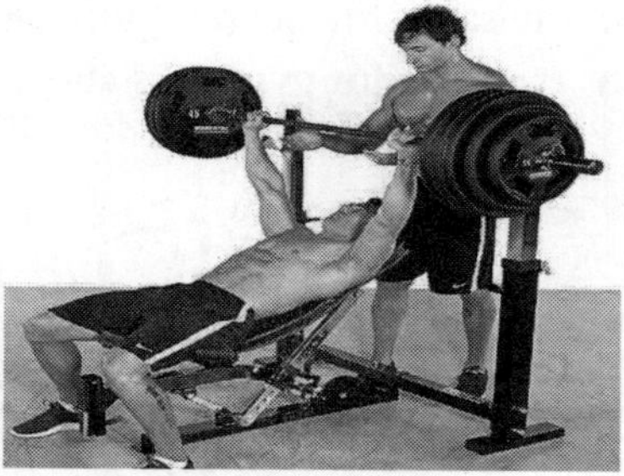

EXERCISE BIKES
Safe if done with proper back support.

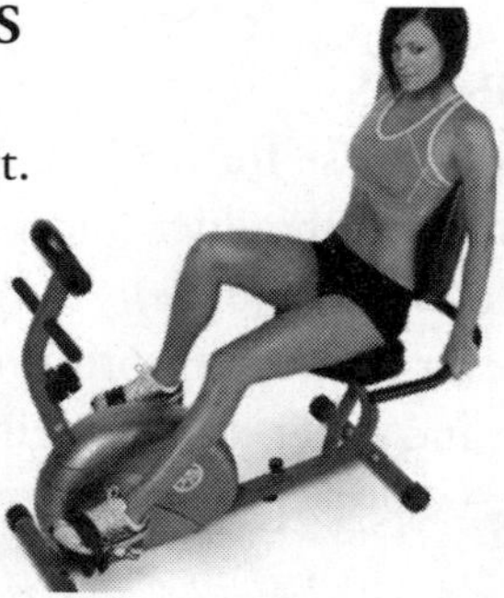

EZ CURL BAR
Good exercise for initial muscle building of upper limb, don't overexert, being regular is key.

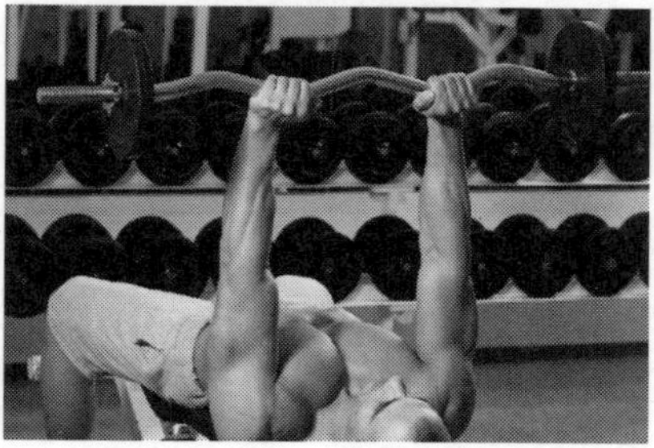

CABLES AND PULLEYS

Dos: Good for biceps and triceps (back of arm) muscles.

Don'ts: Never overdo it, sometimes in weak biceps, this can be ruptured.

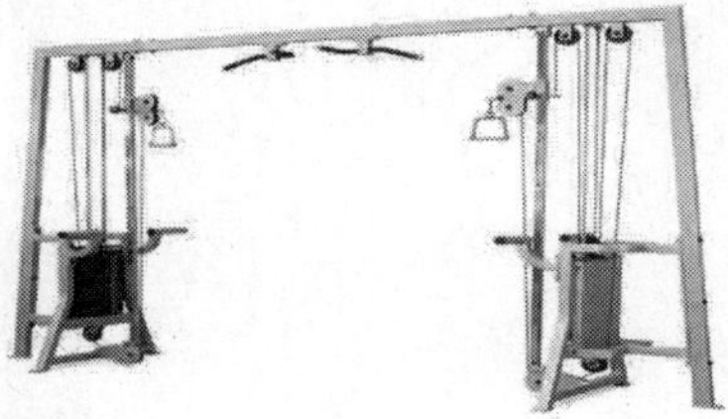

ABDOMINAL BENCH

Dos: Fantastic for abdominal muscles tightening and reduction of pot belly.

Don'ts: Always do in sets of 10 to 15 to avoid risk of abdominal hernia, especially in post caesarean or abdominal surgery patients.

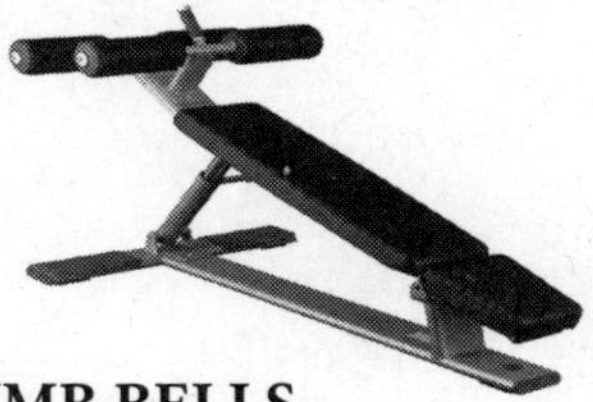

DUMB BELLS

Good for light weight training and build up of muscles of arm.

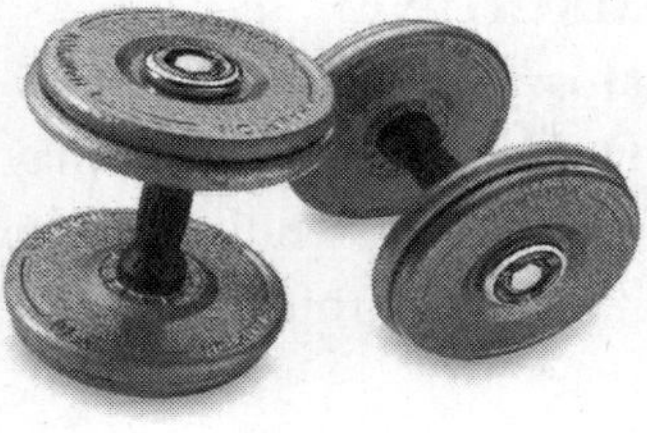

PULL UP BAR

Dos: Strengthening the shoulder girdle muscles.

Don'ts: Risk of shoulders joint subluxation and injury if over enthusiastic.

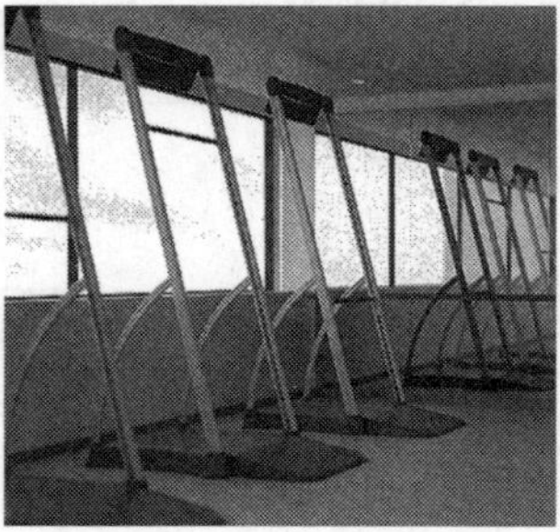

FOAM ROLLER

Dos: Good for body balancing.

Don'ts: People who have vertigo and parkinsonism (brain disease of improper balance) should avoid.

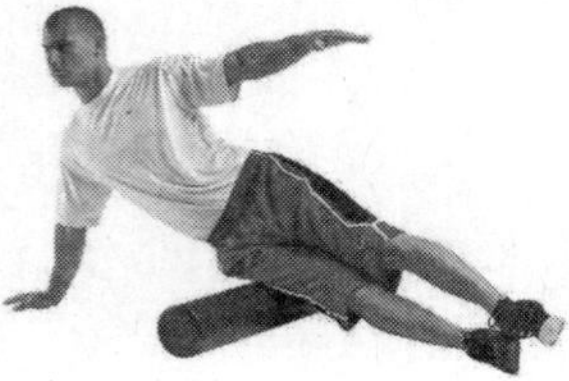

LAT PULL DOWN MACHINE

Dos: Generally safe.

Don'ts: Over exertion may cause rotator cuff tendinitis (shoulder) if done vigorously.

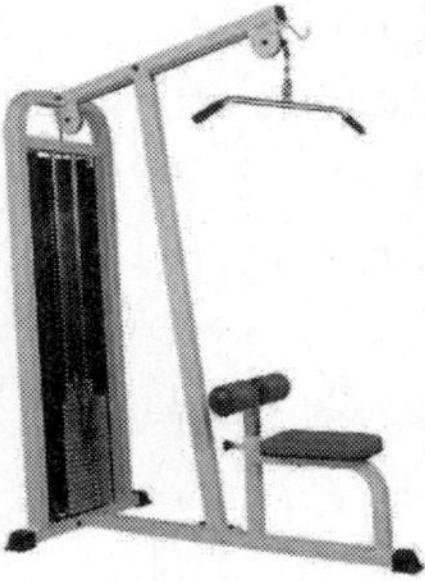

LEG EXTENSION MACHINE

Dos: Good for thigh muscles (front quadriceps and back hamstring).

Don't: Do not increase weight too much, otherwise will affect back negatively; sometimes disc prolapse.

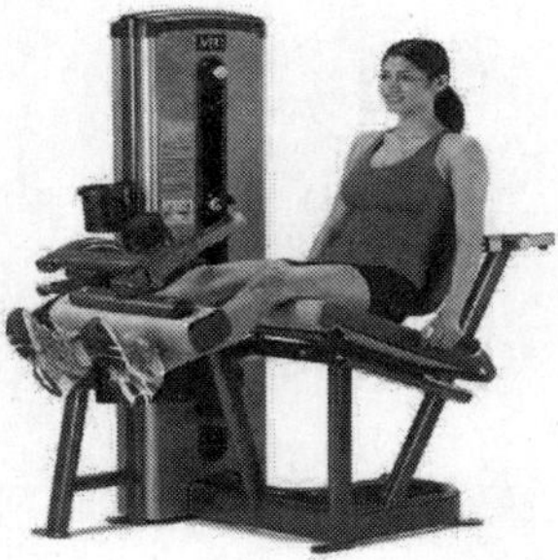

BACK EXTENSION EXERCISING MACHINE

Dos: Regular workout will strengthen back muscles and extremely helpful to fight back pain, especially for office workers.

Don'ts: Aggressive workout avoided in elderly having degenerative changes in spine and excessive forward bending, to be avoided in patients having history of Spondylolisthesis (one bone slipping over other in X-ray).

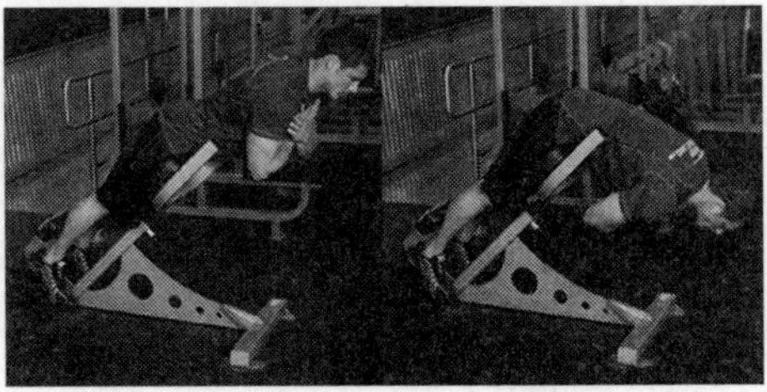